HAVE A MAGICAL DAY!

How to create days filled with calmness and contentment

Claire Reeves

CONTENTS

DEDICATION

This is for you, Andrew - the love of my life. Thank you for being my biggest cheerleader and always believing in me. I wouldn't be doing what I'm doing without you.

And for my beautiful boys, Gethin and Ellis – I hope this helps you to believe that anything in life is possible. Go get your dreams and make them a reality. I couldn't be prouder of the kind, handsome, resilient young men you are becoming.

INTRODUCTION

The fact that you're holding this book in your hands probably means that things are not going so great for you. You want more out of life. You're not on your own with that. The reason I have written this book is that I meet so many people who are stressed out, anxious and just surviving day to day. They believe they can't find happiness until they have got the perfect body, perfect relationship, and perfect job. I think we're all guilty of saying things like..."When I've lost a stone, I'll be happy", "When I am with someone, I'll be happy", "When I'm making better money, I'll be happy". I am here to help you see that without needing to make any big life changes, you can stop waiting for happiness to arrive and create it yourself, with a few tweaks here and there. My mission is to help empower you to take control and truly live a life you deserve. Trust me, life doesn't have to be perfect to be magical.

I love the quote, *'Create a life that you don't need to take a holiday from'*. Again, I hear so many people say, "Only 6 weeks now until I go on holiday, then I can relax and I'll be happy". It is such a shame that life feels so tough, that they are living in the future, wishing the time away to get one week of joy. It's not joy. It's respite from life. Why wait until you go on holiday? You can be happy NOW!

I can honestly say that I love my life and everything in it. I literally cannot remember the last time I had a bad day. I have days more challenging than others but never a 'bad' day. Every day is filled with moments of happiness, love, laughter, learnings and magic. Trust me – I have not always felt like this, (as you will soon see in the next chapter). Even now, I find it harder some days than others to find this happiness. My life, relationships, family and financial situation are far from perfect, but I try to make the best of what I have; change the things that I am not happy with and accept the things I have no control over. No matter how difficult the day has been, I can usually find something positive, whether that be a small act of kindness someone had shown me, like letting me have their parking space or something I can take away as a learning to help me in the future.

Over the last 8 years, I have trained my mind to focus on the good in the most difficult situations or relationships. This has not been easy! And at times, still isn't. I have had to make a complete mental shift, fighting my genetics and ingrained thought patterns, but I assure you, it can be done! I can help you to do this too. Throughout this book, I will tell you what I have learned over the years and help you lighten the emotional load you are carrying on your shoulders. Help you let go of some of the stress and worry that I imagine takes up so much space in your brain. By making some space in your brain, it will allow room to be creative, try new things, re-discover your hobbies and passions and create the YOU that you've always wanted to be.

Anyone that knows me, knows that my happy place is Disneyland. I am a complete and utter Disney nerd! If I was offered a job as a princess in the parade, I'd be there in a heartbeat! I love everything about Disneyland. The colours. The music. The atmosphere. The fun. The wonder. The magic. I remember the first time I went and was completely overwhelmed. I never dreamed in a million years that I would get to go somewhere like that. When I was little, our family holidays consisted of a caravan in a different seaside town in England every year. The highlight was fish and chips on the beach, spending hours trying to win a keyring in the 2p machines.

Don't get me wrong, I have lovely memories of our family holidays, but they were nothing compared to Disney. I was taken aback by how happy the staff were (or seemed! I am not naïve enough to believe that every member of staff sang their way through life after they'd clocked off or that they didn't also have anxieties, money troubles, difficult families to contend with etc.) Every time one of them said, **"*Have a magical day!*"**, my heart melted and I was filled with absolute joy! It is also a place where I can truly connect with the essence of me. On a day to day basis, I'm busy *pretending* to be an adult. Like everyone, trying to keep my shit together, and it is easy to lose touch with who I actually am. At my core, I am someone who is light-hearted; jovial; loves singing and prancing about; loves the Arts and is happy and smiley! Disneyland gets me back in touch with the child in me – the true me.

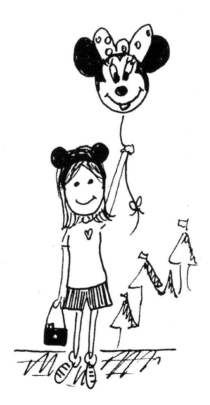

It got me thinking....what if I could re-create this feeling back home? How could I help other people to feel happy, not just when they're on holiday but through all the long, lovely, magical days in between? And so, the writing began!

Now, I am not a writer. In fact, the thought of anyone reading these words terrifies me! However, I will wear my vulnerability with pride and share my story as honestly as I can. I am aware that this completely opens me up to judgment, criticism and perhaps ridicule! The most important thing I have learnt throughout my journey is that if something scares you, it is a sign you need to do it! Without fear and stepping outside your comfort zone you cannot grow. You stay stuck in your old patterns of behaviour and thinking, which probably no longer serve you. I hope that after reading my story, you also gain the courage to push yourself, try something new and show up to the world as who you are. Own your story. Own your quirks and be YOU!

So, without delay, let me tell you a little bit about my journey to happy and how I have learned to make my days magical....

MY STORY

I find it hard to get my head around how much I've changed over the last few years. The person I'm about to describe to you is completely different to the one I am now – it's difficult to believe that that was actually me!

I want to share my journey with you, so that you can see anything is possible! If I can do it, then anyone can!

I have always felt different. Like a bit of a freak, if I'm honest! Growing up, I had fluorescent, wiry, ginger hair and was always by far the tallest in my class. I was hard to miss! I hated everything about the way I looked. I would have given anything to shrink into the background. I longed to be like my friends – petite with brown hair and few distinguishing features. Throughout junior school, I cried myself to sleep most nights wondering what I had done to deserve this curse. Throughout secondary school, I did everything I could to hide and tame my gingerness – from plastering my hair with mousse until it was rock hard and looked like I had been caught in torrential rain, to dying my hair brown which led to many embarrassing disasters.

The worst of these came when I turned up for school looking like a startled, patchy giraffe. My friend came over one Sunday evening to help dye my hair. I had my eye on a boy (which was probably the fourth one that week!) and in my mind, there was no way he would go out with a ginger girl. I had quite long hair at the time that trailed down my back and we had obviously (and quite drastically) underestimated how much dye we would need to cover my thick mane. I remember having my head hanging over my bath, wrapped in towels for protection against the splatters of permanent colour and hearing my friend say, "Erm...I think we might have a problem". We had a massive problem as I realised that the dark, brown dye had barely covered half of my head.

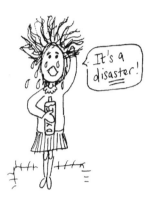

To make it worse, the brown on my head was completely random and patchy. It was horrendous. Of all the nights for it to happen, it had to be a Sunday night when the shops selfishly shut at 4pm. Tears burnt my eyes, as I realised I would have to go to school like that. Shit! Hatred began to race through my veins for my perfectly straight, silky, brown-haired friend who, through gritted teeth, was trying to convince me that it wasn't that bad. Well it was, and I felt like life couldn't get any worse. Part of me was certain she knew what she was doing and had done it on purpose. Now, looking back, I recognise that I was probably being a tad dramatic and that other children have far worse things to deal with, but at that time in my life, my hair was the root of all my pain.

On another occasion, after trying to come to some acceptance of my doomed ginger existence, I thought, "Do you know what...instead of trying to hide my gingerness, I am going to embrace it but I'd be happier if I could just make it a shade darker". So off I went to buy a mahogany dye (being careful this time to buy two boxes) which I thought was going to be the answer to all my prayers. The lady on the box looked happy with her long, flowing auburn hair. Little did I know, that the red in the dye was going to react with the already rouge tones of my hair, to produce what I can only describe as illuminous tangerine. My hair was as orange as a fluorescent highlighter pen. Needless to say, I did not look as happy as the deceitful woman on the box!

I tried and tried on many occasions to get rid of my ginger hair, like it was a stubborn disease. I felt like my efforts were doomed to failure as my bright ginger roots shone through my patchy, semi-permanent dark-brown hair. I looked ridiculous for most of my time at secondary school. As you can imagine, I was bullied every day, usually by some perfectly-formed, blonde-haired, popular girl. I probably made it worse by drawing attention to myself but to me, there was nothing worse than being ginger. Being ginger was associated with being unattractive and no matter what I tried, I couldn't escape it. I hated my life. I hated ME.

I was the butt of everyone's jokes, as boys regularly asked, "Does the carpet match the curtains?" I never did understand why everyone was so obsessed with the colour of my pubic hair. I just didn't get it, but for teenagers it was clearly the height of wit. Once, at my friend's house, his little brother was showing off in front of his friends, thinking he was a comedy genius and he asked me the question. I grabbed him by the hand and said in a serious tone, "You want to see? Come upstairs and I'll show you". He nearly wet himself! The over-confident, brash, 12-year-old almost melted to the floor in a puddle of embarrassment. I did feel slightly bad that I had shown him up in front of his friends, but part of me secretly loved it! I would never actually have gone through with it, but he didn't know that!

As you can imagine, the torture of being ginger and all that came with it, didn't lead to me being filled with confidence. It was completely the opposite. With my friends, I was comfortable – always singing, dancing and being silly. To the point where I was bullied at school by a group of girls who used to write on the tables about me. Beautiful, poetic words such as, 'Claire Collier is a ginger minge'. Lovely! They made fun of me during swimming lessons, they sniggered when I walked past. I didn't know what I had done to make them dislike me so much. I later found out it was because they thought I was too happy with my friends and it irritated them. Bullied for being happy! Crazy!

Communicating with anyone other than my friends though created a state of deep and crippling panic. I was scared of walking down the street in case I had to walk past another person. Walking past a group of teenagers absolutely terrified me, just in case...I have no idea what I thought they might do. I just didn't want people to see me – I wanted to be invisible.

In lessons, I NEVER put my hand up. On every school report it said that I was bright and tried hard but needed to contribute more. I couldn't. Even if I knew the answer to a question, it wasn't worth the risk – just in case I got it wrong and looked a fool! And oh my gosh, if a teacher ever put me on the spot to answer a question, I would literally want to die! I'd be bright red; sweat would pour from every inch of my skin; my eyes wouldn't be able to focus on anything; my whole body would shake, and my heart would be pounding that hard and fast it would take my breath. It crippled me. I was silenced, even though the answer was on the tip of my tongue. I would then spend the rest of the lesson zoned out as I ran the scene over and over and over in my head, calling myself every swear word I knew. This would then haunt me all evening, all night and, if I'm honest, probably for the next few days, weeks and months. I can still vividly remember occasions like this from when I was 10 and I am 37 now!

The worst occasion was when I was in Year 6, the final year before secondary school, and we were in the hall with 2 other classes, playing a game where you had to stand up and talk non-stop about a subject for one minute without saying "Erm". About 5 or 6 children had been chosen to do it and it was horrible. I remember keeping my head down and staring at the rubber-streaked, wooded floor of the hall, hoping not to be picked. It was 5 minutes to 3 and nearly home time, so I thought I had gotten away with it, but to my horror, my teacher, Mr. Lane, said we had time for 1 more and called out my name. I remember my heart physically stopping. I seemed to have lost the use of my legs as I stumbled to the back of the room, trying not to stand on anyone's fingers or trip over their bags. I have absolutely no idea what topic I was given, I just remember not being able to see. Everything was blurred and time seemed to stand still. I must have said "Erm" fifty times and every time, the hall ruptured into cheers and laughter as 90 odd children mocked me for my slip ups. For someone suffering with social anxiety and low self-esteem, this was torture in the purest sense. A memory now firmly ingrained in my brain.

My low confidence really got in the way at times and was a constant frustration. At the end of Year 6, it was tradition for the classes to put on a performance for the parents. That year it was an obscure, musical version of 'Jack and the Beanstalk'. I remember sitting on the floor of the hall as the teachers started choosing who would play which part. Now, as I said, I absolutely love singing and dancing so the initial thought of being part of the main cast really excited me. They wanted the lead role of Jack to be played by a girl and that part involved quite a lot of solos. I desperately wanted it and knew I could be good at it. When the teacher asked for volunteers to audition for the part, a swarm of hands shot up around me but for some reason, I was paralysed. It was like I had a devil and an angel appear on my shoulders. The angel telling me to go for it and put my hand up; the devil telling me not to be so stupid, that I would never get it, that I wasn't good enough, that everyone would laugh at me etc. etc. Anyway, I guess you can imagine. The devil won and I sat in silence, listening to 5 girls sing a few lines from the show, silently judging each one, knowing that I could have sung it better. The girl that got the part then became a constant source of hatred. I hated her. I hated the teachers for choosing her. Really the only person I hated was myself for not having the confidence to go for it but I didn't know that at the time.

As I got older and went to sixth form and university, the bane of my life was introduced...PRESENTATIONS!! My nemesis. My Darth Vader. I think most people are scared of something. Spiders. Snakes. Flying. For me, it was presentations or ANY situations where more than 2 people were looking at me!

I remember being at university and as soon as the word 'presentation' was mentioned, I literally wanted to die. Looking around the room at my classmates, I felt like the only person in the room who was absolutely terrified. Nobody else seemed bothered. I couldn't understand why. For me, there was nothing worse than doing a presentation. I questioned what was wrong with me. I suppose this reaffirmed my dislike of confident people. It took me until I was training to be a counsellor to realise that the hatred I had was because I so desperately wanted to be confident myself. I wanted to be able to talk, be myself and not feel like I was the biggest idiot on the planet. Even being at university as an adult, I scanned down the list of modules and assessments to see the word 'presentation' – my heart stopped. I had an overwhelming feeling that I couldn't do it and, therefore, was going to fail the whole course. It's funny what stories we make up in our heads! I can't put into words how terrifying it was. I think that would be the equivalent now to me jumping out of an aeroplane, but even that I know I could do and still come out of the experience alive!

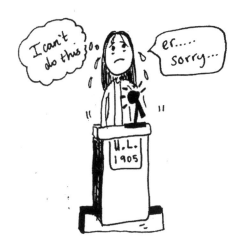

Up until a couple of years ago, I hadn't actually done that many presentations because I was generally 'poorly' on those days! Sometimes, I was genuinely poorly, but the other times, I think I had stressed and worried about it that much that I had made myself poorly. I couldn't understand what was wrong with me. I couldn't understand how other people could talk without their voices quivering or faces going bright red.

Going red for me has always been an issue. I would worry about the thought of going red in front of people which, in turn, made me go red! I wouldn't want people to look at me and feel sorry for me and say, "There goes Claire again - she's really timid and embarrassed all of the time". I hated myself. I hated how I was and I just wanted to be anyone other than me. I noticed the impact of this as I began my career as a teacher. I could deliver an assembly to 250 children and dance and prance about with not a care in the world, but as soon as one member of staff came into the hall, I would feel the heat rise in my face, my anxiety would be triggered, which paralysed me.

I don't think my lack of confidence was helped by the way I was brought up. Don't get me wrong, I love my parents and I don't blame them because I know they did their best. My mum completely wrapped me up in cotton wool and instilled in me that the world was a scary, dangerous place. As a little girl, I cried everyday not wanting to go to school, teachers had to drag me off her. I was completely traumatised at the thought of being separated from my mum. Anybody else scared me. Life scared me. My dad on the other hand was very harsh and critical. I always felt that I wasn't quite good enough and never quite met his expectations. I always did really well at school and got mostly As on my reports. If I got a B in a subject (which was probably Science) my dad would focus on that and want to know why it wasn't an A. I think because I was quite a sensitive soul and already didn't like myself, any hint of other people thinking I wasn't good enough was exaggerated and I took it to heart. I've always just felt that the way I looked, the way I was, everything about me wasn't what I wanted it to be and wasn't quite good enough for everybody else.

As a child, I literally worried about everything. I worried about handing in my homework. I worried about my hair. I worried about what everyone else would be wearing. I worried about what was in my lunchbox. I remember my Year 6 teacher calling me 'a worrier'. I just thought that was who I was. I was a worrier and I couldn't do anything about it. There was nothing anyone could do or say to stop it. That's just who I was and I had to deal with it.

Growing up, I didn't really have a role model or an example of someone who wasn't like that. My parents were both very anxious, pessimistic people, always waiting for something bad to happen. To the point where, I was brought up thinking that if an ambulance went past, then that it obviously involved someone in our family and it was normal behaviour to ring everyone just to make sure they were OK. How crazy is that?? It was only up until a few years ago that I thought that was completely normal! Everyone in my family is exactly the same. That way of thinking was engrained in us. I honestly didn't realise that I could be any different.

My pessimism wasn't helped by my parents' difficult separation when I was a teenager. For five years, they split up and got back together, desperately trying to find a way through the mess that was our family. This was an incredibly difficult time for all of us; it felt as though it was never-ending. For years, I would start the New Year thinking, "It's going to be a good year this year". It never was. The hurt and drama continued for ten years, until I got pregnant with my first baby and miraculously out of nowhere, my parents decided that they could be civil with each other after all. I had been let down so often by my parents and their crazy situation, I felt that I was never going to be happy. I couldn't ever let myself get excited about anything because ultimately our plans would be ruined by their drama. I couldn't even get excited about my honeymoon, as I just presumed that I wouldn't end up going as something would inevitably go wrong. I worried about everything and anything and was constantly scared about the future.

The point where I realised that something had to change was when I got a job working for the council. A few weeks after I started, the organisation was restructured, and I was told my job was changing and that I would have to reapply for it. The new job included organising and leading meetings with professionals and parents. If this had been in the original job description, then there would have been absolutely no way on this planet I would have even considered it! But I needed a job and I had only just started there, so at that time I didn't feel like I had any other choice but to go for it. I thought, "How on earth am I going to be able to do that when I can't even speak in front of a couple of people without getting flustered, going red and being a blithering idiot?" So that was when I went for CBT. I think I only had 4 or 5 sessions. We looked at where the thoughts and beliefs about myself had come from. The therapist set me homework, which was to talk to myself in a mirror, record myself talking and ultimately film myself so that I could see what I looked like when I spoke in front of people. Oh my God! I could not do it!! I just remember laughing in the session and thinking, "You're an absolute plonker to suggest that. Why would I record myself and watch it back?!" That to me was insane! Torture! How would that be helpful?! So, in the end, I made up some silly excuses about why I couldn't go to the sessions anymore. I think I blamed it on childcare issues! But it had worked a little bit. I got the new job, started leading the meetings and although I was nervous, pushing myself to do it and facing my fears did make me better at it.

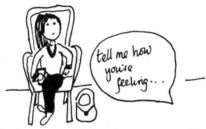

My mood and the way I felt about myself drastically took a turn for the worse when I had a baby. It has taken a lot for me to admit that I found having children immensely difficult. I always thought that my purpose in life was to be a mum. I had visions of me being this perfect mum, who baked cookies and made creations out of toilet roll tubes, but I quickly realised that being a perfect mum wasn't as easy as I thought. I spent every waking minute trying to figure out how to master this 'mum' thing and be better. I had spent my life working hard and being a high achiever, so I couldn't understand that even though I was trying harder than I had ever tried with anything, I still wasn't getting it 'right'! I couldn't deal with it. I had always been so in control and organised so that I didn't fail - this was something I felt like I was failing at on a daily basis because every time the baby cried, I felt as though it was evidence that I wasn't doing a good enough job. I ran through the checklist in my mind. Does he need changing? Feeding? Is he tired? Has he got wind? After I'd been through the checklist and done everything I could think of, the only thing left to blame was me. I must have been doing something wrong.

I tried so hard with my first baby to meet his every need before he had the opportunity to cry - he never had to try for anything or wait. He had everything he needed, wanted and more. I found every day incredibly tough and couldn't see what I could change to make me a better mum.

He wasn't much of a smiler (which in my mind was more evidence that I wasn't making him happy). I spent hours every day jumping around, pulling ridiculous faces, pretending to fall over to make him smile, often to no avail. This frustrated the hell out of me. I wondered what was wrong with me that I couldn't even make my own baby smile. Even at times when I thought I'd cracked it, he would go through phases of teething or get poorly and the routine that I had worked hard to instil went out of the window. I felt like a failure all over again.

On top of this, my old insecurities came flooding back. Not only was I ginger and unattractive but now I was fat and ginger and, in my eyes, just hideous. My confidence was at rock bottom. I constantly worried to my husband's dismay that he was going to leave me for someone else. I didn't understand why he would stay with me. I was fat, ugly and useless at everything.

Not only was my mood and confidence low but my anxiety was ramped up to a whole new level. I lived with a constant panic that something was going to happen to my baby. I felt out of control and like I didn't trust myself. I had regular disturbing visions and nightmares of something terrible happening, like me leaving the bath water in and him drowning in the night; looking out of the window to see him falling and hitting the ground; that I'd look in the back of the car and realise I'd left him in his car seat somewhere. I felt like I was losing my mind. I was overwhelmed with anxiety.

By the time my second baby came along, it just all got too much. I couldn't meet his needs as quickly as I would have liked as I also had a demanding toddler to contend with. I just felt like I was doing a shit job! I was struggling. Ultimately, when my second baby was about one, I was diagnosed with depression. I felt I had a good understanding of what depression was as I had done a Psychology degree and witnessed my parents struggling with their mental health, but little did I know! It completely shook my world. First of all, I didn't understand how I could be depressed, as at the time, I was training to be a counsellor. Surely that would mean I wouldn't be a very good counsellor if I couldn't even manage my own emotions? Again, this was just more evidence that suggested I was a massive failure. I just couldn't shake it off. I had everything I wanted: two beautiful children; an amazing husband; we'd recently moved to the house of my dreams; I'd had a brand-new car for my birthday. I literally had everything I could possibly want. I had a family and friends that loved and cared about me, yet I felt alone and completely empty. I didn't feel like I knew how to be happy anymore. I felt miserable, but most days I just didn't feel anything which scared me even more. I felt like I was bringing everyone down - a burden. I felt like people would have been better off if I wasn't there, as I was an ungrateful, miserable, selfish brat.

Fortunately, I have never felt suicidal, but feeling those feelings of wanting to get away terrified me and shocked me into getting some help. I needed to get myself better for the sake of my family. I took myself off to the doctors and was prescribed anti-depressants and referred for counselling. This coincided with me spending time with my husband's cousin, Jenny, who had recently discovered meditation and the Law of Attraction. This really opened my eyes to a new way of thinking. From there, the journey to my recovery and self-discovery had well and truly started! I made it my mission to get well and learn everything there was to know about positive thinking and improving mental health. I completely immersed myself in this world and tried everything I could to get myself better, to feel more positive and more in control. This continues now, every day.

So, that's me. You may be able to relate to some of my story. You may not. That's ok. I just want you to understand that we all have a story. We all have a past, but we don't need to live there. We don't need to do the things we've always done; believe the things we've always believed. We are free to be who we want, and we can reinvent ourselves as many times as we need, to become a version of ourselves that we are happy with. Own your story, accept it and let's look at how we can start creating your future...

This book is a collection of all the things that I've tried over the last few years. Being the inherent perfectionist that I am (or was!), I initially made the mistake of trying to do everything all at once. I was then burnt out from positivity! I suggest that you try one thing at a time to see what suits you. It is worth trying everything once so that you can then see what works for you and which things you would like to adopt into your life.

A word of warning though...

This is the start of something very exciting for you as I'm going to teach you a completely new way of thinking and being. However, your life isn't going to change overnight. As you would go to the gym to train your body which can take months, if not years, to get it to where you want it to be, training your brain is very similar. It's going to be challenging at times as it requires a complete mental shift, but if you commit to applying these strategies consistently, I guarantee that you will see an improvement.

As I said at the beginning of this chapter, my life has dramatically changed for the better over the last few years. Don't get me wrong though, things aren't perfect. I still lose my way, have the odd meltdown, crisis in confidence and my old patterns of thinking emerge from time to time. This is natural and I try not to beat myself too much when this happens. The beliefs I had about myself and the world had been with me for a long time, making them hard to shift. It's especially easy to fall back into those unhelpful patterns when I'm run down or stressed. Anxiety and low confidence are apparently still my default settings. This happens far less than it used to though. I can usually spot the signs when I'm falling back into the hole and now have the tools to get myself out of it much quicker.

I'm now at a point where I like myself. I'm mostly happy with how I look (there may be bits that I could improve but I try not to focus too much on those!) and 99% of the time I can confidently say that 'I am good enough'. I have had the confidence to make some quite big changes in my life, such as leaving my very stressful job and setting up my own, successful counselling and coaching practice. I have created a life that works for me and my family. I now set my own working timetable, I see friends, spend time with family and have rekindled hobbies that I am passionate about. I have two happy, beautiful children and an incredibly supportive and handsome husband, without whom none of this would be possible. I'm truly living the life of my dreams. You too can have this! If you change your mind set, you can change your world, and bring magic to your days.

So, now it's over to you. I wish you all the luck in the world as you discover the beauty of life and the beauty of YOU!

BEING AWARE

The first step of any journey is the hardest. Admitting you're not happy; admitting you're struggling and you need help is the hardest, yet most important part. It is much easier to plod on from day to day, hoping that one day things will get better. It is easier to think that when I have more money, things will get better; when the children start school, I will have more time; when I've lost weight, I'll be happy. Why wait until that happens? You can be happy NOW! Your happiness and contentment with life is not dependent on other things and certainly not on other people. Happiness comes from you. This is your life. Do not wait another day.

You might be thinking...if it was only that easy! I appreciate that you may have had a difficult start in life; you may have had controlling parents; you may have experienced abuse. I imagine you have had something in your past that you've struggled with that has knocked your confidence or faith in humanity. It may have shaped your beliefs about yourself to the point where you now feel that whatever you do in life isn't good enough, or that you're not important, or that you don't deserve love or happiness. Or simply that the world is a bad place. This is not the truth. You have learnt these beliefs through things you've been through, things you've heard others saying or by picking up unconscious signs. You weren't born believing that you weren't good enough. Think back to when you were two or three years old – you thought you were the bomb! You weren't lacking in confidence then! You didn't care what people thought. You thought you were amazing as you twirled around in your princess dress or fought imaginary super-villains. You were unstoppable.

So, what I'm saying is, if you've learnt to believe these negatives things about yourself and the world around you, surely you can unlearn them and learn a more positive, healthy, empowering way of thinking? Of course you can...and in the next few chapters I am going to show you how.

Take control of your life and your happiness TODAY!

You can do this.

I believe in you.

HOW TO USE THIS BOOK...

I've attempted to cover everything I've learnt over the last few years and divide them into five sections to make it easier to digest. Everything is connected – mind, body and spirit. It would be unrealistic to expect to feel good just by relying on positive thinking. If you don't do any exercise and you regularly abuse your body by eating high-calorie foods, smoking and drinking alcohol, then there's bound to be a negative impact on your mental health and how you feel about yourself. If you feel rubbish about yourself, then this can impact all other areas of your life – relationships, confidence at work, etc. You need to focus on you as a whole person. On all five areas.

As I mentioned earlier, I wouldn't recommend you try all of the suggestions in the book in one go. The good thing about this book is that you don't need to read it from cover to cover. You can dip in and out of it as you see fit. I would probably read a section at a time and just pick a couple of things that you fancy trying and do them every day until you notice a positive difference. Have you heard of the 21/90 rule? If you do something every day for 21 days, it becomes a habit. If you do that thing for another 90 days, it becomes a permanent lifestyle change. It takes time but it'll be worth it.

Equally, you might try something and find that it really is not for you. That's absolutely fine. Please do not use this book as another stick to beat yourself over the head with! Out of all of the things I am suggesting, I now only do a few of these but I have stuck with the things that have made the biggest difference to me. I get up at 5am; exercise first thing in a morning for at least 30 minutes; I don't eat meat or dairy (other than the odd bit of cheese!); I meditate and practise gratitude every day; I set myself regular goals which I put on my bathroom mirror and I use visualisation and the power of the Law of Attraction to bring positive things into my life.

You have to find what is right for you.

SO, LET'S GET STARTED...

I believe that the formula for changing your life and bringing magic into your days lies in getting the balance right in the following areas, which I have called the 5 Cs.

1. Challenge your thoughts
2. Control your emotions
3. Compassion and confidence
4. Care for your body
5. Create your future

CHALLENGE YOUR THOUGHTS

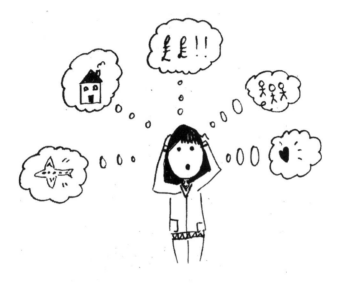

"Your calm mind is the ultimate weapon against your challenges."

Challenge Your Thoughts

Did you know that we think between 60,000 and 80,000 thoughts every day?! That's on average about 3000 every hour! Our mind is constantly active, flitting from one thing to the next, never staying still. Our thinking is an automatic process, as automatic as breathing and blinking and is something we have little control over. If you suffer with anxiety, this constant stream of thinking is exhausting, as you over-analyse and over-think everything. That's what anxiety mostly is though... thought. Thoughts about the future, thoughts about bad things happening, thoughts about things going wrong. If we can learn to manage our thoughts better, then we can control how we feel and act. What we think, affects how we feel, which then affects our behaviour. Identifying the thoughts that lead to anxiety is a brilliant first step in managing it and decreasing the symptoms. See the following cycle...

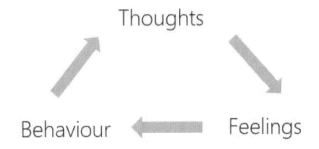

Take the following example...

Your new work colleague asks everyone in the office if they would like a hot drink, but she misses you out. You interpret this situation with thoughts that she obviously doesn't like you. This then triggers feelings of anxiety/insecurity/frustration/confusion and because you think she doesn't like you, you find yourself behaving differently around her - you're quieter and try to avoid her where possible. This then means that you never really get to know each other and therefore that initial thought of never disappears. If anything, the change in your behaviour and the fact that you haven't built a relationship confirms that initial thought of, "She doesn't like me".

Can you see how easy it is to get stuck in this loop? This section will help you to identify negative thoughts so that you gain control over them and choose what to do with them.

Observer to your thoughts

It's important to understand, that you are not your thoughts. Let me say that again...YOU ARE NOT YOUR THOUGHTS. You don't have to listen to them or act on them. They are not always real or a true reflection of reality.

Don't believe me? Just start to notice your thoughts and the stories your brain tells you on a daily basis. It may tell you a story, convincing you that you should not try that new exercise class because people will laugh at you; not contact that friend because she's obviously annoyed with you as you haven't heard from her for a few days; your partner is losing interest in your as they were a bit off on the phone! Your brain jumps to these conclusions as it's job is to protect you and scan for potential danger. It wants you to be tucked up at home on your own, away from everyone and everything: that way you are safe! It's a worried aunt that much prefers you didn't get a life at all.

Noticing your thoughts is the first step to putting you in control. It helps to create distance between you and them. It makes you realise that they are not YOU after all. One of the first books I read on my journey was, 'The Power of Now' by Eckhart Tolle. This book changed my life. It made me realise how much my behaviour and emotions were governed by my thoughts. The moment I realised that I didn't have to listen to the thoughts in my head, was the moment I realised that I did not have to be controlled by my anxiety. That I could control it.

Have you ever just stopped and listened to the thoughts that pop up into your head? I think you'd be surprised by how random they are! But also, how constant they are. One minute you will be thinking about what you are going to eat for tea; then you'll be thinking that you need to nip to Sainsbury's to get a prize for the children's school fayre; then you'll be worrying about your little boy being behind in his reading; then you'll be thinking about how much you loved school as a child; then you'll be thinking about secondary school when you were bullied...the train of thought just rumbles on and on. It's not always a pleasant journey. Your thoughts can kidnap you. Steal you away from real moments that matter. But you can fight back. Would you like to learn how to step off this train?

A simple exercise is to close your eyes and just notice your thoughts. Notice them with curiosity and without judgment. Don't try and control them. Just go with it and see what pops up. Imagine yourself sitting on a riverbank next to a babbling brook. As the thoughts pop into your head, imagine putting them on a leaf and watch as the leaf floats past you on the water. Don't try and stop the leaf or pick it up, just notice it floating by. Say to yourself, "Isn't it interesting that I am thinking about what my friend said to me yesterday...what I am having for tea...about the presentation I have to do next week." Just observe. Some people find it helpful to imagine their thoughts as a separate little person in their head, a little negative chatterbox! Again, it helps to create distance between you and your thoughts so that you can consider whether you are going to listen to them or not. You are not your thoughts. You can choose.

If you are a worrier, like I used to be (and still am at times), you may find that a lot of your thoughts are very negative and can feel intrusive. They feel overwhelming and lead to anxiety, which for some people, triggers panic attacks. Although our thoughts are mostly random, they are also there as a protection mechanism, warning you of possible threats. Your brain is a very clever device. It wants you to stay alive. However, most of the time we're not in danger, but our brain doesn't know that. It still operates in caveman mode. You see, thousands of years ago, humans lived in the wild, surrounded by the constant threat of being eaten alive by some terrifying pre-historic creature. Our brains therefore had to be skilled at scanning for danger in order to protect us and stay alive. Even though we do not have sabre-toothed tigers freely roaming our streets, our brains haven't lost this incredible hyper-sensitivity to our surroundings when it believes there's a threat. It is always looking for things to go wrong - this is known as 'negativity bias'.

However, our biggest threat in the modern world is other humans - worrying what they think about us; worrying about them having better things than us; worrying about the comment they made on Facebook and whether it was a dig at us! The thing is, the chatterbox in our head sometimes gets things wrong. As it tries to predict what's going to happen to help us, it can tell us things that aren't necessarily true.

For example, I met up with my friend and I noticed that she wasn't herself. She kept looking at her watch while we were having a coffee and I found it really off-putting. An hour had passed, and she said she needed to get going as she'd got lots to do. I felt really disappointed by this as I had expected to spend the whole day with her. After she left, I felt really deflated and couldn't help but feel that she didn't want to be with me, that I wasn't interesting enough or that I had upset her in some way. The chatterbox in my head taunted me with negative thoughts all day, to the point where I'd dramatically made my mind up that we could no longer be friends and that I wouldn't bother getting in touch again as I obviously wasn't a good enough friend. Later that night, after I'd spent an hour ranting to my husband about it, my friend text to apologise for leaving early and explained she couldn't settle as she was waiting for her mum to call with results from the hospital, with the possible diagnosis of breast cancer. I felt like an absolute fool. Of course, she'd have been looking at her watch. Of course, she'd have wanted to get home. I felt silly that it hadn't occurred to me that there could be another reason. This is what our brain does – it tries to make sense of things by filling in the gaps but it's usually with negative things.

So, when my brain goes to this place now and the Chatterbox in my head is warning me about something, I say, "Thank you for trying to protect me but there is no threat" or "...thank you for the warning brain but right now I am OK." I might ask myself, "Is this just a story I am telling myself or do I know this for a fact?" It's OK to listen to the thoughts but they don't need to change your behaviour and get in the way of you doing things.

You might find though, that your mind starts to kick back and throws up the "...yes, but, what if...?" If you hear this, be very aware! 'What if's...' are very dangerous creatures! Once you start with the 'what if's', it can quickly spiral out of control and before you know it you have told yourself a whole story about what MIGHT happen. The crazy thing is, you actually convince yourself this is what is DEFINITELY going to happen. Sound familiar to you? Listening to your thoughts about what *might* go wrong is a waste of time and energy as we have absolutely no way of predicting the future and we have absolutely no control over it. If you start to notice these 'what if' thoughts, then just gently bring your attention back to the present and remind yourself of this – "I cannot predict the future. I have no control over it. I only have control over what I do and how I feel now."

I wonder...could you change the 'what if' predictions into something positive happening?

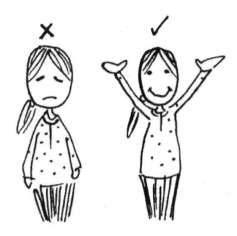

"A negative mind will never give you a positive life."

Question your thoughts

So, you receive a message over the weekend from your boss asking if he/she can have a meeting with you on Monday morning. You've convinced yourself that you must be in trouble and you're in for a telling off. Next, you've told yourself the story that you're going to get fired...then you're not going to be able to find another job because no-one will employ someone who has just been fired...you won't have enough money to pay the bills...so you will lose your home...this will put strain on your relationship with your husband, so you'll get a divorce...you'll be depressed...turn to alcohol...and will be living on the streets for the rest of your life! All because your boss has asked to speak to you! Now, I know I'm not the only one who does this! It is exhausting!

The best way to stop this train of thought is to get off the train! Challenge these thoughts and ask yourself, "What evidence have I got to support the thought that my boss is unhappy with me?" You might find that you haven't got any evidence to support this. Then ask yourself, "What evidence have I got against this thought?" For example, your boss seemed OK with you on Friday when you left the office; even praised you that day for a report that you had handed in before the deadline; you've never been in trouble before; you're conscientious and always put 100% of effort into your work; if you have done something wrong then it would be a genuine mistake.

Then ask yourself, "What else could she want to speak to me about?"' I am sure there are a million other things, most of which could be positive. Remember: your brain is always trying to prepare you for the worst to protect you. However, it's so not helpful! When you start challenging your thoughts, it can be really helpful to write them down so you can clearly see the evidence 'for' and 'against'. When you're used to doing this, you'll be able to do this in your head much easier and faster. You could draw yourself a quick chart that looks something like this...

Evidence to support the thought	Evidence against the thought	What else could I think?

Remember...you can't stop your thoughts, but you can choose whether to pay attention to them or not. Your thoughts are not always real!

Is this within my control?

Whatever it is that you're worried about, ask yourself, "Is there anything I can do about this now?" or "Do I have the power to control this?" If the answer is 'no', then worrying about it isn't going to stop it from happening or change the situation. Another thing to ask yourself is, "Is this worry productive or unproductive?" Quite often, what we're worried about tends not to happen anyway, or it's never as bad as we imagine it will be. If you ask yourself those questions, and the answer is 'yes', then think carefully about what your next steps need to be. It might be helpful to write down the possible steps you could take or talk these through with someone you trust. If it is within your control and you *can* do something to alleviate some of the anxiety and stress you're feeling, then you must take action. Putting it off and trying to push it to the back of your mind doesn't work. Take control. Sometimes all it takes is for you to have a conversation with someone to help put your mind at rest and the weight of worry is lifted. Talking really does help. A problem shared is a problem halved.

If your problem or worry is something like, "I'm not sure what will happen if..." or "What happens if I get there and can't find my way...", try and find out as much information as you can beforehand to help put your mind at rest. Think to yourself, "Can I find out the answer to this question?" If you can, then doing a little bit of research can really help to alleviate your anxiety.

Here are a few examples of things that are not in your control:

- What other people think
- How other people behave
- How other people feel
- What happens in the future
- What has happened in the past

- Life!

Things within your control:

- How you respond to situations
- Your emotions
- Your behaviour
- What you say to yourself in your head and the stories you tell yourself
- How you respond to other people's emotions
- How you interpret other people's behaviour
- How you respond to your thoughts
- Who you choose to spend your time with
- How you choose to spend your time
- Asking for help when you need it
- The amount of action you take towards meeting your goals
- Your self-care (diet, exercise, personal hygiene, taking time to relax)
- Putting your needs first
- How many times you smile today!

Remember...you are only in control of you.

"When the sun shines in your eyes, remember you control your eyes, not the sun."

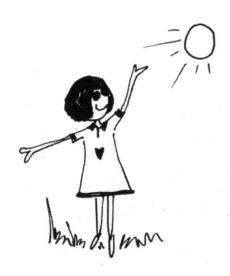

You are not a mind-reader!

In situations that scare us, we tend to go into mind-reading mode, imagining what people are thinking and what they are saying about us. I must admit this is something that I still catch myself doing on occasion. It drives me insane.

I find it particularly hard to charge clients a cancellation fee. My policy is that if cancelling within 48 hours you pay 50% of the session fee and if cancelling within 24 hours then you pay 100% of the fee. I am getting better at this as I understand how important clear boundaries are in the work I do. Also, I am running a business that is helping to provide for my family. However, this situation completely triggers my anxiety. After I have sent the text informing the client that they will have to pay a fee, my negative Chatterbox runs riot. It will run through the following statements a fair few times, in between obsessively checking my phone for a response!

Your client will think…

…"you're horrible!"

…"you don't care about them and their situation."

…"it is unfair and they're going to complain about you."

…"you're money-grabbing and greedy."

…"you're rubbish at your job and that they won't bother booking another appointment again."

This goes on and on until I eventually hear back from the client who usually says that they completely understand and transfer the fee.

The negative Chatterbox appears elsewhere too. I love dancing and joined an adult street dance class. It was mainly the mums of the children who did the junior classes. We had been practising all year and it was time to perform at the Christmas Showcase. Many of the other mums that performed were worrying about what others would think - maybe they looked like an idiot, they were too old, they were an embarrassment, they were too overweight to be dancing. Let me ask you this...if you saw a group of women on a stage performing a street dance – what would you think? I can't imagine your first thoughts would be any of those things. I imagine you'd think how brave they were and how you wish you could do something like that.

When you find yourself mind-reading, ask yourself this, "Do I know for a fact that they're thinking this? What else could they be thinking? What would I think about someone else in this situation?" I have learnt that we can NEVER know what's going through someone else's mind, so there's no point in trying to guess. When we guess, we often get it very wrong! We don't know for definite that people think we're stupid, ugly, fat, scruffy, uneducated (or whatever other horrible things we say to ourselves). They could be thinking how happy we look, how they would like a round bottom like ours, what pretty eyes we have or where we got our shoes from! We always default to the negatives and discount the positives. Remember your thoughts aren't real. They're just your brain's way of flagging up threat. Other people's thoughts and opinions of us are not dangerous though. We don't need to let them have an impact on how we feel about ourselves.

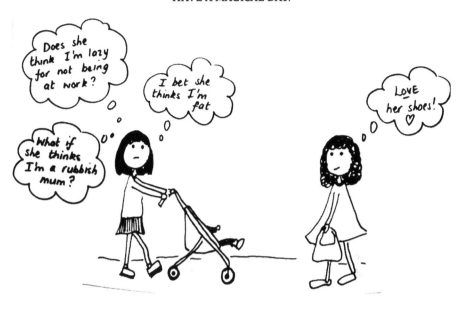

Remember...you are not a mind-reader!

Mindfulness

So, you've decided there's nothing you can do to change or control the thing that's playing on your mind. How do you stop those thoughts from coming back and interfering with your day? The answer is...you can't! You can't stop your thoughts, but you can try and gain control over them. You may have heard about mindfulness? Mindfulness is the psychological process of bringing your attention to the present moment and being fully aware of what you're doing or what's happening around you.

This practise can really help to get these anxious, negative thoughts under control. As they start to creep back in, without judgement, gently push them away and bring your attention back to what you're doing. It can be helpful to practise this when you're not stressed, that way, when you are stressed, focussing on the present will happen more naturally and will help to alleviate some of the anxiety you're feeling. This is like any new skill that you learn – it takes commitment, patience and lots of practise.

A simple exercise to start with could be to practise being mindful when you're washing the dishes. I absolutely hate this job, and I know that if my mind is going to wander, it's going to be when I'm doing this!

• Start by running the water and listening to the sound it makes as you fill up the sink.

• Watch as the bubbles start to form once you've put the washing up liquid in.

• Move your hands in the water, notice the temperature and what it feels like on your skin.

• Pick up each dish individually and carefully wash away the dirt, being mindful to remove every last bit.

When you're first starting out, it can be helpful to talk to yourself in your head and create a running commentary of what you're doing. For example, "I'm picking up the red bowl and wiping it with the yellow sponge to clean off the Bolognese, which I must say was delicious!" The more you're talking to yourself, the less chance the negative thoughts have of making an appearance.

Another exercise is mindful walking.

· Start by walking with your head held upright and not looking down at your feet.

· Feel connected to the Earth by noticing what every step feels like.

· Notice the speed in which you're walking.

· Shift your attention to each foot, as your feet take it in turns to lift from the ground.

· Notice how your weight shifts from right to left, left to right.

· Look around you and notice your surroundings with curiosity. What wildlife can you see? Are there any interesting buildings? What can you hear?

· Notice the breeze on your face and breathe it in slowly and deeply.

· If your mind is wandering, count each step or repeat a simple mantra to yourself in time to your steps. For example, 'I...AM...PRESENT' or 'I...AM...CALM' or 'ALL...IS...WELL.'

Remember...the only thing you have control over is the present moment.

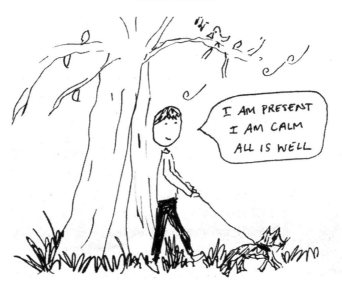

Give your brain a break

One of the best ways that I've found to give my brain a break and be present is by doing jigsaws! You can't possibly focus on the negative thoughts spiralling in your head while you are focussing on searching for the pieces. There's nothing more satisfying than putting a piece in the right place. I feel a sense of pride and accomplishment (maybe a bit over the top, but you know what I mean!).

Some people find that doing word searches, sudoku, Candy Crush or crosswords have the same effect. Adult colouring books are becoming more popular as a way of relaxing and switching off from a busy day. Sometimes we just need to stop and get off the anxiety merry-go-round – this is perfect for that! I wonder what you could try to give your brain the well-earned break it needs?

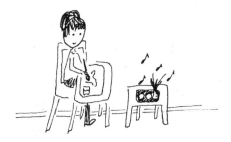

Remember...it's just as important to rest your brain as it is your body.

Attitude of gratitude

So, we're aware of our thoughts now and have realised that they are mostly negative! Our brains are definitely built for survival not happiness! How do we go about taking control of our thoughts and changing them to more positive ones? There is no better way to start the day than by getting yourself in a positive mindset, by expressing gratitude and appreciation for everything you have in your life. It is easy to focus on the negative, what we don't have, what is going wrong in our lives but, how much time do we spend focussing on everything we do have? Gratitude is such a powerful emotion. Research conducted by Dr. Seligman, a psychologist at the University of Pennsylvania, has shown that people who express gratitude daily are generally happier.

Research conducted by the National Institute of Health uncovered that people who regularly expressed gratitude had higher levels of activity in the hypothalamus, which is the part of the brain that plays a part in regulating metabolism, sleep and stress levels. Other research conducted by the UCLA's Mindfulness Awareness Research Centre found that gratitude literally changes the molecular structure of the brain, can boost the release of the neurotransmitter serotonin and activate the brain stem to produce dopamine, both of which are chemicals known for increasing feelings of happiness. It has also been noticed that people that practice gratitude generally have healthier relationships, increased resilience, increased self-esteem, sleep better, exercise more, experience less pain and have lower blood pressure.

Starting your morning with an attitude of gratitude, will set you up for the rest of the day. A brilliant way to get this started is as soon as your alarm goes off, say, "Thank you!" You have been given another day! No matter how tired or run down you feel, before your feet hit the floor, say to yourself, "Thank you Universe. Today is going be a great day." Even if you feel the opposite, say these words. Repeating positive mantras helps to start retraining your brain by creating new positive neural pathways in your brain. So, just as you would exercise your body regularly to keep it fit, you need to do the same to your brain to keep you mentally fit. Say "Thank you" with every step you take to the bathroom and repeat the phrase above while you're brushing your teeth. Before you've gone downstairs for breakfast, you've already set yourself up to be in a positive mood.

Remember...start your day as your mean to go on!

Gratitude journal

A great way to bring gratitude into your daily routine is by writing in a daily gratitude journal. A gratitude journal is simply a diary of things that you are grateful for. While you're eating breakfast, before you go to sleep or at any point in the day when you need a wave of positivity, write down three things you're grateful for in your life. It could be people, material things or experiences you've had. After you've written each one, take a moment to close your eyes and really feel that gratitude in your heart. Let it fill your chest until it feels as though it could burst with love.

Write something different every day. The idea is not to repeat anything in your journal and after a few days you'll start to find it difficult to think of new things to be grateful for. You'll have written things like, "I'm grateful for my husband, my children, the house we live in, my job, my car..." and then you'll really have to start thinking about the things we all take for granted, such as, hot running water, having a toaster or having electricity. You will be forced to open your eyes and physically look for positive things. You may start to notice how beautiful the flowers in your garden are, or how incredibly beautiful the clouds look in the sky. The small things will really start to matter.

Your daily gratitude practice can involve others, which can be beneficial for your relationships. Writing thank you messages on post-its, sending a thank you card, writing a gratitude letter or sending a text can really mean a lot. You'll feel great for your act of kindness and expressing how you feel, and you never know, you may receive thanks and kindness in return.

The practice of gratitude can really start to improve how you feel, simply by shifting your focus onto positive things. Studies by Emmons and McCullough (2003) found that participants that kept a journal of things they were grateful of were more optimistic, exercised more and had fewer signs of illness. They also reported an increase in mood, enthusiasm, determination and alertness. They were also more likely to help others and make progress towards their personal goals than the participants that didn't keep a journal.

You can buy gratitude journals online or you could just get yourself a little notebook – you don't need anything fancy. If you love stationery as much as I do, this may be an excuse to treat yourself to a swanky new notebook that you can fill with all things positive! Some people find it beneficial to incorporate this into their daily morning routine, others find it more beneficial to just write in a journal once a week. Find what works for you by giving it a go. This practice for me, along with challenging my thoughts, has been the most beneficial thing to helping me with my mood and anxiety.

Remember...no matter what the situation, there will always be things to be grateful for if you look hard enough.

Gratitude stone

There are many other ways you can bring gratitude into your life. While you're out and about mindfully walking, appreciating the nature that surrounds you, find a small, smooth stone. You can then keep this in your pocket so as you're queuing in the post office or waiting in the playground to pick the children up, you can hold this in your hand without anyone noticing and it will be a reminder to be grateful. I wrote, 'Thank you' on mine and decorated it with a permanent pen, but again, you don't need to. I also had one in the change part of my purse, so that every time I opened my purse to pay for something, it reminded me to be grateful for the money I had.

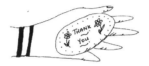

An area that I have started to become interested in is the healing powers of crystals. Rose Quartz is perfect for practising gratitude as it is known for its healing heart energies, helping to release emotions of unconditional love, restore trust and harmony in relationships and promote feelings of peace and forgiveness. Holding a piece of Rose Quartz whilst thinking of the things you are grateful for would be a perfect addition to your daily positivity practice.

I wonder...what you could do to remind you to be grateful?

"Every day may not be good but there is good in every day."

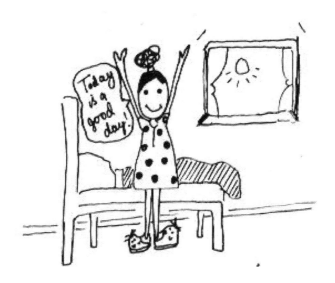

Positivity bracelet

As we know, our thoughts create our emotions. Our negative thoughts are usually intrusive and automatic. To become more aware of our thoughts and create distance between us and them, it can be helpful to wear a bracelet/bobble/elastic band on your wrist and every time you think a negative thought, swap it to the other wrist.

I have heard of people wearing things on their wrists and twanging them to cause pain as a distraction from their thoughts and feelings. What I am suggesting is not about causing pain. You are merely moving the bracelet to raise your awareness and gain a sense of control over the thoughts. If you hear yourself worrying about something, putting yourself down or complaining about something or someone – stop and be aware. Once you raise your awareness, you can pause and then choose what you fill your head with. Are you going to listen to the negativity in your head or are you going to choose to think and believe something else?

I still wear my bracelet every day, but now it's just a reminder to stay positive and to choose happiness.

Remember...your goal isn't to get rid of negative thoughts; it is to raise your awareness to them so that you can change your response to them.

The Law of Attraction

Even though we have talked about your thoughts being the main culprit of anxiety, if utilised in the right way thoughts can be your most powerful tool to help create the life you want. Thoughts are energy, and whatever you think about will be attracted to you like a magnet, according to the Law of Attraction. So, if you regularly think negative thoughts, you will attract negative things into your life and if you regularly think positive thoughts, you will attract positive things into your life.

When I learnt about this theory and started thinking more positively about situations, people and experiences, I noticed that positive things did start happening. I have always stressed about money and when I have worried that we haven't got enough or have been waiting for something to go wrong, it inevitably has - the car would break down or I'd get a big bill that I wasn't expecting. However, when I started to change the way I thought about money, practised gratitude for the money I did have and believed that the Universe would provide me with abundance, I would get an unexpected cheque in the post; opportunities at work would come up for me to earn more money or I'd get discount in a shop that I wasn't expecting.

A simple example of this force at work is when patients take placebo drugs to cure an illness. Research has shown that patients taking the placebo drugs, made the same amount of progress as patients taking the actual drugs. If you believe something will work, then it usually does. The power of positivity can be truly amazing. After learning about this theory, I guarantee you won't believe in coincidences anymore. The Universe is always at work, leaving us little signs and getting things in order for us. It's like magic!

So, how does it work? The Law of Attraction works like ordering out of a catalogue. Once you have placed your order, you expect that you will receive that thing. Place your order to the universe (no matter how big or small the things are) and wait for the magic to happen. I typed out my 'order' of things I wanted to attract and put it on my bathroom mirror so I could see it day and night. On my list I had things like a new car, a new TV, for my husband to get a promotion, for me to have 'x' number of clients. I wonder what you would have on your list to the Universe and what you would like to attract into your life?

Once you have your list, when you wake up in a morning and before you go to sleep at night, close your eyes and picture yourself having these things. Feel the emotions that you would feel if this was your reality, if you had already received these things. Really feel as if it's already happened. You see, your brain doesn't know the difference between reality and the imagined. If your unconscious mind creates a belief that something has already happened, it will quickly attempt to validate it as being true. It will find evidence to support this new belief which helps you to become aware of new opportunities that positively impact this belief. Your behaviour and thought patterns will shift also, accommodating this new belief. Things start becoming aligned and the thing you most want is drawn closer to you. I think a lot of it is to do with the power of positive thinking *and* making physical changes to achieve what you want to achieve but sometimes the Universe works in mysterious ways and it really can feel like magic!

Let me share with you my magical story…

We had not long moved to a new house and money was tight. I was only working a few hours each week as the boys were little. We had had to borrow a lot of money from family (and various credit cards) to be able to afford the move. It didn't help that we were in negative equity. We were desperate to get ourselves straight and back to being financially comfortable. We worked out that we needed £20,000 to pay off everything we owed regarding the house; change our battered car and pay off bits of finance we had, like our sofa etc. £20,000 was the magic number. I wrote it out on a blank cheque along with my name and I stuck it next to my bed. I looked at it day and night, imagining a whole scenario where I was handed this cheque. I imagined I had won it in a competition or by playing the lottery. As soon as I started to focus my attention on attracting this money, I started noticing 20ps wherever I went. I lifted the rug to hoover and I found one there. I emptied the washing machine and there was one sitting in the bottom. I found them in my shoe. They were everywhere - it was getting spooky. At one time, it was getting that ridiculous that I accused my husband of planting them!

Once I was ironing, turned my head to look at something, looked back down at the t-shirt I was ironing and there was a 20p on top of it, just staring back at me. I was the only one in the house and I had absolutely no idea how it got there. I must admit, that freaked me out slightly! I was finding that many that I started saving them and before long I had a hefty chunk of change. I was starting to feel like the Universe was sending them to me – 20 was my magic number after all, just with a few less zeros! Over the next year, many things happened...the boys and I were involved in a minor car accident and we all received compensation; my husband had been offered a second job and earned quite a bit of money from that; we had a tax rebate that we weren't expecting; we had PPI money that added up to quite a bit. All in all, in 1 year, we had received (almost to the penny!) an extra £20,000 that we hadn't planned for and weren't expecting. It might not have come in the lump sum that I had imagined but it came! Thank you Universe!

You may feel sceptical but try it, you'll be amazed! I test it sometimes by asking the Universe to save me a parking space outside the shop I am going to. As I am driving there, I visualise the space I want and 9 times out of 10, it's there waiting for me or someone is just pulling out of it.

Practising gratitude is another way to start attracting positive things into your life. If something does go wrong, like you're stuck in a traffic jam, ask yourself, "What can I learn from this?" and, "What is positive about this situation?" Being late for things used to drive me crazy with anxiety, now I say "Thank you Universe" and think, "At least I'm safe sitting in the car. If I wasn't here, maybe I could have been in an accident further along the road. Thank you Universe, for protecting me."

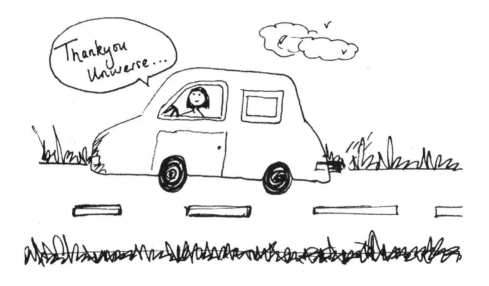

If you look hard enough, you can find positives in most situations. The more you practise asking yourself these questions, the easier it will become and good things will start to happen. There are no such things as coincidences – everything happens for a reason! If you want to find out more about how you can start attracting positive things into your life, read 'The Secret' by Rhonda Byrne.

Remember...thoughts become things. If you can visualise it, you will attract it to you.

Are your beliefs holding you back?

Every second of every day we are processing billions of pieces of information through our five senses. It is thought that we have to ability to process eleven million pieces of information per second unconsciously, while consciously we process approximately forty pieces per second. So, what stops all this information from entering our conscious mind? This is something known as the Reticular Activating System (RAS) which acts as a filter for our five senses. It only lets information through that it thinks are significant and of interest to us. It shows us information that is in line with what we focus on the most. If we have negative beliefs, it will show us proof that back these up.

Imagine what life would be like if we didn't have this filter. Our brains would be likely to explode with the overwhelming amount of information. Without this filter we would find ourselves having to process everything as if it was the first time we'd encountered that thing. We would constantly have the need to re-learn everything.

The RAS has three ways of breaking down the information into more manageable chunks for us:

It **deletes** – it just gets rid of or ignores information that it doesn't think is relevant or important. If your brain didn't do this, you'd be overloaded.

It **distorts** – it twists information to fit in with what we believe, it makes global misrepresentations of the information. For example, if you are scared of snakes, a piece of rope lying on the floor in the distance may be perceived as a snake to fit in with what your brain wants you to focus on. It is great at helping you to survive and looking out for potential dangers.

It **generalises** – it put things and experiences into groups and makes global conclusions. For example, if you've been nervous speaking in front of people before in a meeting at work, your brain will generalise all meetings as anxiety provoking situations.

The problem is that, because of the RAS, you are not always getting an accurate picture of experiences, people or of yourself. Isn't it interesting that if ten people witnessed a crime, every one of them would have a different account? This is because they would have been focussing on different things, things that were more important to them.

The information we receive is filtered based on our beliefs and values. Our beliefs act as a lens of which we see things through. These beliefs are formed usually between the ages of 0-7 years, known as the imprint period. This is when we start to get a sense of who we are, what we're good at, what we're not so good at, who we can rely on, whether the world is a safe or scary place. The beliefs we have about ourselves can be formed by something as simple as comparing ourselves to our siblings and other children at school. Comments from our parents, grandparents, teachers can all add up to build a picture of who we are.

I remember when I first started in Year 6, our teacher had asked his previous class to say a few words summing up what they thought out about each of us, his new class. Goodness knows why he felt that sharing this with us was a positive thing to do. He went down the list of names saying things like, "Ryan – you're funny, sporty and a really fast runner", "Amy – you are quiet, kind and good at reading". When he got to my name he said, "Claire – you look down on others"...and then just moved on as if nothing had happened. In that moment, I felt crushed. Children that I'd never even spoken to before had the impression of me that I looked down on others. This couldn't have been further from the truth. I was painfully shy and quiet at school, but I kept myself to myself and as far I was aware I got on with everyone. Still to this day, I wrack my brains wondering what I must have been doing for them to get that impression. From this I developed the belief that I wasn't likeable and I know that that one comment has shaped who I am today. I spent the next however many years, trying to please people. Going out of my way to be extra kind, extra nice and extra self-deprecating, I imagine to avoid people thinking that about me again. It's taken me a long time to shift this belief and stop worrying about what other people think of me.

Let's explore this a bit further and look at how beliefs are formed. Take the belief, 'I'm not good at art'. Tony Robbins explains that the formations of beliefs can be likened to a table. Over time, we experience situations that contribute towards the growth of the belief and if you imagine each situation to be like a leg of the table. It could be that a friend laughs at your drawing at school (table leg number 1); a few years later, you show your mum a picture you have drawn and she squints as she tries to figure out what it is, which makes you feel bad (table leg number 2); you look around you at school and realise your artwork is not as good as the other children's (table leg number 3) and then to confirm this, you get a 'C' on your school report for Art when all of your other grades are 'A's (table leg number 4). It only takes a few experiences to start building a firm belief. The belief is then held up like a sturdy tabletop. Once its been formed, it sticks.

The beliefs we have can have a massive impact on our lives as they unconsciously drive our behaviour and our responses to things. When our beliefs are negative, they can limit us and the decisions we make. These are called limiting beliefs. As I've said previously, your brain filters information to fit in with what it thinks is important to you. Even though the belief is negative, your brain will actively find information and evidence that fits with this. We are creatures of habit and we like things to be predictable. An example I use to explain this is the reason why people stay in unhealthy relationships. Even though the relationship is toxic and unhealthy, the predictability of the unhealthiness becomes safe. This can feel less scary than leaving and finding a more positive relationship. We want to know where we stand. We want certainty.

Let's take this scenario...

Simon has developed the underlying belief that, 'I will be rejected'. He feels upset when his wife goes out with her friends and feels incredibly jealous when she talks to other men. He finds himself becoming distant from her leading up to the day when she is due to go out. He is snappy with her and questions her when she gets back about who she's been speaking to. His wife feels as though he doesn't trust her, and this puts a strain on their relationship. His wife has never given him any reason not to trust her, but Simon finds evidence. He checks her phone regularly and often reads into things that aren't there. Simon is not proud of his behaviour and consciously tries to convince himself that his wife loves him and that she won't leave. The underlying belief is powerful though and by filtering the information before him, he can make information fit into his belief. He can find proof.

This is what we all do. We ignore the positives that go against that belief and just focus on anything that fits with what we already believe. For Simon, there might have been a big long list of things that his wife had said and done to demonstrate her love and commitment to him, but Simon's brain ignores these things and focusses on the one thing that proves she is going to leave, like her being 10 minutes late home or not kissing him good night.

A perfect way to illustrate this selective attention and our ability to filter information is 'The Invisible Gorilla' experiment. You can find this on YouTube or www.theinvisiblegorilla.com. I won't say anymore because I don't want to give anything away!

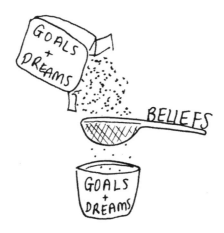

Remember...our perceptions and memories are based on information that has been filtered. They are not necessarily a true reflection of reality.

"What consumes your mind controls your life."

Positive self-talk and affirmations

Another way that you can start to drown out the negative Chatterbox is to immerse yourself in all things positive. Find positive quotes to stick on your bathroom mirror, on your fridge, on your desk, etc. The more you read these, the more ingrained they'll be in the new positive pathway in your brain. I have a little book in my car that has 365 positive quotes, so whenever I'm stuck in traffic or if I arrive early for an appointment, I can open it and read a few while I am waiting. Knowing that I'm using that time to my benefit makes me feel great and in control.

Google Images, Instagram and Pinterest are amazing for finding great quotes and affirmations. I've even printed some off that I like, along with the lyrics of Robbie William's 'Love My Life' song, and put them in frames in my bathroom so that I can read them as I am getting ready in the morning and last thing before bedtime. My go-to affirmation is, 'I have enough. I do enough. I AM ENOUGH', as I regularly need a reminder of this.

So, what exactly is a positive affirmation? A positive affirmation is a statement or mantra that you say to yourself repeatedly that helps to challenge negative thoughts, limiting beliefs and raise self-esteem. They help to re-program your unconscious mind. Basically, you tell yourself what you most need to hear. If there is an area that you are struggling with, for example, confidence then your affirmations will centre around that. For the affirmations to work, you need to consistently repeat them at least 3 times a day until you start to believe them. Imagine they are like exercise for the mind.

Here are a few examples:

I am confident at expressing my emotions.

I am enjoying the challenges of my new job.

I trust myself to make decisions that are right for me.

I am important and put my needs first.

When writing your affirmations, they need to be personal to you, they need to mean something and feel emotive. Here are some other tips:

- They can sometimes feel more powerful when they start with the words, 'I am...'
- They need to be in the present tense, like they are already happening, or you already feel this way.
- They need to be positive and affirm what you want, not what you don't want.
- The shorter and simpler they are, the better, as you are more likely to remember them.

Sometimes, if you have a really stubborn limiting belief, like 'I am not good enough', telling yourself, 'I am good enough' may not work as well because your unconscious mind will just reject it. If you find that your affirmations aren't having the desired affect and after a few weeks, you still cannot consider adopting them as part of your new belief system, then it's sometimes useful to play around with the wording of them. My hypnotherapist gave me some great advice and helped me to make my affirmations less direct. She explained that if they are worded in a gentler and less obvious way, then the filter to your unconscious mind will sometimes miss them and allow them to pass straight through.

Try beginning your affirmations with the following...

I am finding ways to...

I am allowing myself...

I give myself permission...

I am choosing...

I give myself the freedom to...

I have had an ongoing battle with self-care and at times have run myself into the ground by focussing on what everyone else needs instead of my own needs. I have repeated the affirmation, 'I am important' for years but it has never really gone in. When I changed the wording to, 'I am allowing myself time to relax', and, 'I am choosing to consider my needs first', it made all the difference. My behaviour started to change in line with these affirmations and I started to believe them to be truthful.

Affirmations can also be useful to help you manage your emotions in certain situations. For example, if I had to do some new training, I might feel quite nervous and my self-doubt would no doubt creep in. To combat this and keep me calm, I would repeat something like this to myself..."I am confident. I am capable. I am calm." I would repeat this over and over in my head to drown out the self-doubting, self-sabotaging voice. You can say whatever you need to hear. Imagine if you were giving a friend a pep-talk, what would you say to them? Give yourself that same kindness and compassion.

Positive self-talk is so important to overcome anxiety and to feel better about yourself. It is important to listen to the names you call yourself and the negative things you say. I imagine at times you are guilty of saying things like, "Why did you do that, you idiot?", "You can't wear that, you look fat", "You just made yourself sound stupid". Imagine if you had a person following you around all day saying those things to you. I'm not sure it would make you feel great and I am not sure you'd want to stick around. You are doing this to yourself. Ask yourself, "Would I say these words to my children/partner/best friend?" If the answer is no, then don't say them to yourself. Try this...

for every negative thing you say about yourself, replace it with 3 positive affirmations and you'll soon notice the difference.

Research has been done by IKEA to test the power of positive words using plants. Experiments were set up with two plants. One of the plants was spoken to in a critical, bullying, insulting way and the other plant was spoken to using positive, complimentary, encouraging words. After 30 days, the plant that received the insults had droopy leaves and looked a tad dishevelled. The plant that received the compliments was thriving and had fuller, healthier, deeper green leaves. If words can have this much impact on plants, imagine what they can do to humans.

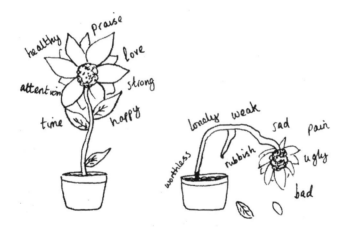

A similar experiment was carried out by Japanese researcher, Dr.Emoto, using rice. He placed rice into three glass containers and filled them with enough water to submerge the it. To the first container, he said, "Thank you." To the second container, he said, "You're an idiot", and he ignored the rice in the third container. After a month of repeating these phrases daily, the rice that was thanked fermented and smelt pleasant. The rice that was insulted turned black. The rice that was ignored began to rot. Dr. Emoto explains how important it is to consider how we are treating people and the words we are using, as they have a powerful affect.

Remember…talk to yourself like you love yourself. Positive words encourage growth. Negative words literally destroy and rot.

N.E.T. Time

It is as important to feed your mind a healthy diet, as it is your body. We all need downtime and a little light relief from the daily stresses, but we can quickly get sucked into the habit of doing the same thing every night – sitting on the sofa and watching TV. I think most of us are guilty of putting the children to bed or coming home from a hard day's work and settling down in front of the TV, only to rise to re-fill our cup of tea. Conversation can be limited, with couples sitting on different sofas watching mind-numbing reality TV shows or separately scrolling on devices. Like I said, this is perhaps OK every now and again but what else could you be using that time for?

That's where N.E.T. Time comes in. It stands for 'No Extra Time'. It's about consciously filling your mind time with positive, uplifting content that will challenge your thinking and help to improve your mental health. I understand how hard it can be to find the time to fit in exercise, never mind thinking about your fitting in a healthy mental diet as well. N.E.T. Time helps you to find those precious minutes that could be helping you to move forwards in your life, towards your dreams and goals. All it takes is for you to think outside the box about where you could find space in your day. It might also be worth considering how you could adapt your evening routine for it to be relaxing but also be moving you closer to where you want to be.

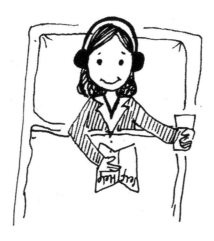

There are so many things you can do in your N.E.T. Time to help you grow more mentally fit. It could be listening an audio book, a TED Talk, podcast, video on YouTube or reading a self-help book and you don't need to make extra time for these. You could be listening to these while you're cooking, ironing, walking the dog or driving to work. You could be reading whilst waiting to pick your children up from their afterschool club or waiting for your dentist appointment. The time is there if you want to find it.

Remember...the more positivity and learning you can squeeze into your days the better, as this is all necessary to re-wire your brain to start thinking in a new, healthier way.

You are an adult!

There are many modalities of counselling and one that has helped me to overcome my anxieties within relationships is Transactional Analysis. Learning the basics was all I needed to help me challenge my thinking. It is thought that each individual has three ego states or parts of our personality. Three states that are triggered when we have interactions with others. The ego states are Parent, Adult and Child.

The **Parent** ego state is what we might find ourselves going in to with our own children. Have you ever heard yourself say something that your parents used to say to you? Whenever we are thinking, feeling and behaving in a way that is a copy of what our parents did, we are in our Parent ego state. This could be in a critical or nurturing way.

The **Adult** ego state is when we are thinking, feeling and behaving as we would in the present.

The **Child** ego state is when we are thinking, feeling and behaving as we would have done when we were children.

When we are interacting with another person, depending on what ego state they are communicating from, it can trigger one of our ego states. For example, I know that if I spoke to someone who came across as stern and critical, I would automatically find myself feeling and behaving like a nervous child as they would probably remind me of my dad.

A few years back, I had a manager who was lovely but was known for having quite unpredictable moods. Unpredictability in people is something that really triggers my anxiety – I like to know where I stand. Whenever I had to knock on her office door to ask her a question, I would instantly turn into a child and feel flustered. I would stutter when I spoke and feel about an inch tall. I used to walk away from her office feeling like a complete idiot and often thinking, "What is wrong with me?!"

The way I combatted this was by repeating the following with every step I took along the corridor to her office – "I AM AN ADULT! I AM AN ADULT! I AM AN ADULT!" When I got to her office, I made sure my body language reflected that of a confident adult, instead of terrified child. Needless to say, this had a massive impact on our relationship. A small change in my communication style led to a change in her. She started communicating with me from an adult place instead of that of a critical parent. Over time, I felt a shift - within our relationship we had become equals. Two adults. Our communication improved significantly, and she actually became a good friend of mine, as well as my boss.

Remember...you are an adult!

Different model of the world

Another way to change your focus and include more positivity in your life, is to accept that everyone has a different model of the world. Even if you completely disagree with the way someone behaves, it doesn't necessarily mean it is wrong. They have just developed a different view of the world because of their upbringing, personality, values and beliefs. They're simply following a different script. Just because someone behaves badly, it doesn't mean that they are fundamentally a bad person. People are not their behaviour. Shift your focus. What is good about this person? What can you be grateful for?

If I came across someone driving erratically or an angry driver in the car park in Sainsbury's on a Saturday afternoon, I always ask myself, "I wonder what could be going on for that person?" The erratic driver could just have received a phone call that his wife has gone into labour and he's in a rush to get home. The angry person in the car park could have just had a bereavement and is picking up flowers to give to a family member. Try to open your mind to other possibilities. Try and find the positives.

Remember...things are not always black and white.

Forgiveness

It's easy to blame others for the way our lives have turned out, especially our parents. We might believe that they didn't show us enough love; they put us down; they favoured our brother/sister; they loved us too much and smothered us. There is no such thing as a perfect parent. For a long time, I blamed my parents for my lack of confidence and low self-esteem. However, over time, I've learned that they did their best with the emotional and material resources they had at the time. You can continue to live your life carrying your past around with you and have it weigh you down, or you can forgive. Forgive doesn't mean forget, but it helps you to lift blame and negativity and helps you to take control of your life.

My parents are great, but they have not always handled things as well as I needed them to due to them having their own struggles. I'm now grateful for the hard times we have been through and I'm grateful for them as people - complete with their interesting quirks! If it wasn't for my parents, I wouldn't be the person I am today. I wouldn't be writing this book, that's for sure. Because of how I was raised and what I went through in my childhood, I had to develop empathy and put others first. I had to develop an understanding of other people and be able to read their moods and emotions. This may sound awful but I've learnt to be a good mum by doing things differently to my parents. My relationship with my husband is open, honest and strong as I have learnt the importance of being a unit and not working against each other, like my parents did. I thank my parents for all my struggles.

Once you start seeing your parents as ordinary people that have their own story and personal struggles, you can start to remove some of the blame. I love the affirmations from Louise Hay's deck of 'Power Thought Cards'...'*I have compassion for my parents' childhoods. I now know that I chose them because they were perfect for what I had to learn. I forgive them and set them free, and*

I set myself free.' I love the idea that we chose our parents as they were the best people to teach us what we needed to learn.

I wonder...what positives can you take from having the childhood and parents that you had?

Take responsibility

Removing the blame from your parents and practising forgiveness only really leaves you with one option, and that is to start taking responsibility for your own happiness and ultimately, your own life. Listen to yourself as you talk to others – do you constantly blame other people and things for what goes wrong in your life? Do you make excuses as to why you can't do certain things? Do you constantly compare yourself to others and say things like, "Well, it's OK for them because they have..."? You may have been through a tough time; you may not have had the best start in life, but that doesn't need to stop you from creating the life you want now. Life is short and can change in an instant. If you want something, go out and get it! If you want more money, what can you do about it? If you want to be thinner, what can you do? If you want to be happier in your relationships, what can YOU do?

Where would your behaviour fall on the diagram below? Above the line or below the line?

Ownership	Accountability	Responsibility
Blame	Excuses	Denial

**Remember...you cannot change other people,
but you can change yourself.**

There is no such thing as failure

I have never been very good at failing! The first time I failed something was my driving test when I was 17. I have always been conscientious and when I've tried hard at something, I've usually achieved well. I tried so hard with my driving but still failed – how did that happen? My test had gone well until I nearly hit an old lady on a pushbike, who looked as though she'd had too many brandies, swerving in and out at the side of the road! I have hated pushbikes since then!

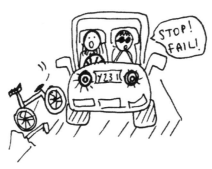

If things don't quite go to plan, then we tell ourselves that we have failed; that we could have tried harder; that we could and should have done better. Failure is something that most of us fear and that drives a lot of our behaviour. However, *there is no such thing as failure, only feedback.* Take the pressure off yourself. Remind yourself that *you have not failed; you just got a different outcome than what you expected* and now you have information that can help you to succeed in the future.

From my driving experience, I quickly learnt that sometimes things are not within our control; I learnt to always give cyclists more room as you pass them; I learnt that I need to respond assertively and always signal to the other drivers what I am about to do. I now believe that the Universe provides me with opportunities to learn. Maybe that day I needed to learn more about other road users to prevent me from having an accident in the future. The Universe will keep putting obstacles in your way until you have learnt the lesson from it.

The next time something doesn't quite work out the way you wanted, ask yourself, "What have I learnt from this experience? What can I take from it?" If you have learnt something, then the experience can't be all negative.

Remember...resilience is the key to success. Pick yourself up and try again with your new-found knowledge.

Life is change

I used to spend my life worrying about tragedies befalling me or my family. Accepting that bad things WILL happen, and that life is change really helped me. This is one of the key principles of Buddhism. I have learnt to accept that life is going to throw up difficult situations, but that doesn't mean that I have to let them affect my mood, stress levels and relationships. I've accepted that the good, but more importantly, the bad times do not last forever but that bad things ARE going to happen. Life is pain and suffering. Once you accept this, it can relieve some of the anxiety you feel.

Anxiety is predicting what will happen in the future. If you already know that the future is going to hold bad times as well as good, then why wait for it? You know it's coming, it's just a question of how you handle it when it does come. One thing I have found incredibly helpful, is repeating to myself daily that, "I can handle anything". I know I can! I've been through tough times and I'm still here, stronger and wiser than before. I know that nothing lasts forever. A few years ago, things like my car breaking down would have completely stressed me out. I probably, would have thought, "Why do these things always happen to me?"

The way I handle it now is by having gratitude for having a car in the first place and for appreciating all the miles the car has allowed me to travel. I think of all the amazing places those tyres have taken me; the friends they've allowed me to see and how much easier my life has been having a car and not having to rely on public transport. I'm grateful for the bill! You can fight against the suffering and get angry or simply accept it for what it is.

**Remember...you can handle anything
if you find the positives.**

Pull out the weeds!

Changing the way you think is the first step to freeing yourself of anxiety and other negative emotions. However, realistically you can't just rely on the power of your thoughts and the power of the universe to get things done for you. Positive thinking and visualisation (which I will cover in 'Creating your new life') speed up the process of helping you to make changes, but there needs to be more. ACTION! I love Tony Robbins' analogy of a garden. He says that if you walk into your garden and it's overgrown with weeds, you can't just tidy the garden by optimistically thinking, "The weeds will go. The weeds will go. The weeds will go". Tony says, "You need to get into the garden and pull up some f**king weeds!"

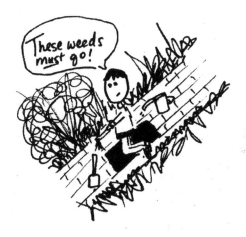

Remember...positive thinking + action = big changes!

In summary…

To change the way you think is going to take time. It certainly isn't going to happen overnight. The more you challenge your negative thoughts and look for the positives, the easier it will become, as every time you learn something new, new neural networks are formed in the brain. The more you practise this way of thinking, the more engrained these new pathways will become, and your brain will just automatically go there.

Imagine an ice skater skating round and round the ice rink, carving a new path into the ice. Once that path is carved, it's very difficult for them to change directions as their skates just want to follow the grooves. It's the same with your thoughts, they want to follow old patterns, old pathways. It's time to make some new grooves! Some new, positive grooves that help you to grow instead of holding you back. I am not the same person I was 8 years ago; my brain really is wired up differently and yours can be too. Just be consistent, patient and **you will get there.**

CONTROL YOUR EMOTIONS

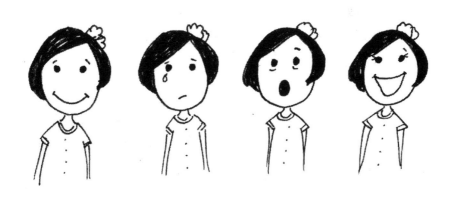

"Inner peace begins the moment you choose not to allow another person or event to control your emotions."

Control Your Emotions

What are emotions and what are they for? Emotions are psychological and physical responses to a particular event. The main emotions we experience are: joy, surprise, fear, disgust, anger and sadness, but we also have feelings like jealousy, frustration, nervousness, disappointment, excitement and determination. The emotions we feel have an impact on our behaviour and the day-to-day choices we make; they help us to express ourselves; to be understood by others; motivate us to take action and help us to survive by responding to threats. However, as helpful as they can be, too much of any of these emotions can leave us feeling out of control.

Emotions are useful as they are indicators and messages that perhaps something isn't right, but they're not always a true reflection of the situation. Our emotions can feel exaggerated at times. Our emotions are often triggered by our thoughts, which are triggered by our model of the world and how we perceive it. Two people can experience very different emotions about a situation depending on their previous experience, core beliefs and values. However, whatever you are feeling cannot be wrong. Don't let anyone tell you that. It is your truth. Only you can decide whether how you feel is real or whether your emotions are being triggered by something else.

Choose your emotions

This is the single most life-changing lesson from my own counselling. To be told that I was in control of how I felt, absolutely baffled me! My family are all worriers and are very pessimistic, glass half-empty sort of people. This is how I was and how I thought I would always be. I had no idea that I had the power to change that.

Have you ever started your day by stubbing your toe or spilling coffee down your shirt before you were about to leave for work? I imagine that you said a few naughty words and it may have put you in a bad mood. Have you ever noticed that if you've started the day feeling negative then more bad things happened? I'm sure you've even said, "Oh great, it's going to be one of those days!" Wouldn't it be great if you could stop this chain of events and no matter what happened, had a good day? Well, you can! Whatever challenges you face, you can choose to be annoyed, frustrated, angry, sad or you can choose to focus on the positives and what you have learnt from that situation. Sometimes you have every reason to be upset. Allow that emotion in, feel it, accept it, but then you don't need to let that one thing spoil the rest of your day. Choose to move on. Choose to be happy! I start every day by telling myself that, "No matter what happens, I am in control. It's going to be a good day!"

As I've said, you choose how you feel. No-one else has the power to make you feel anything. Again, learning this, blew my mind! Guilt was my life. I constantly tried to please people and worried whether I had upset someone or let them down in any way. I often said the words, "She's *made* me feel really guilty". That's the thing though - nobody can *make* you feel anything. Nobody has that much power that they can control your emotions.

Take the following scenario...

You've arranged to meet your friend for dinner. You get home from work after a stressful day, with a banging headache. The last thing you feel like doing is going back out. All you want to do is get in your pjs and lie in a dark room. You text your friend an hour before to explain that you feel unwell, apologise and ask if she would mind rearranging. Your friend immediately texts back, "OK (no kiss!)." You get the feeling from her reply that she's annoyed.

You now have two choices:

1. Let the feelings of guilt wash over you. Beat yourself up about what a bad friend you are. Send a long, rambling text message back, apologising profusely. Let this ruin your whole evening and probably make your headache worse. Worry about what you are going to say the next time you see her and rehearse this conversation a million times.

Or...

2. Ask yourself, 'Have I done anything wrong? Have I been out of order? AM I A BAD PERSON?' Hopefully you answer 'no' to all of those! Accept that you are not in control of your friend's emotions, only your own. Send a short message back saying, 'I will be in touch to rearrange soon. Would love to see you x'. Leave it at that. Put your pjs on, get into bed and nurse your poorly head, feeling content that you've put your needs first and are doing your best to take care of yourself.

I think this is a really important point to reiterate.

You are only in control of your emotions. No-one can control your emotions. You cannot control anyone else's emotions.

In that scenario, you can choose to feel guilty and upset, or you can choose to be happy and content. Equally, your friend could choose to be annoyed and upset or she could choose to be a little disappointed, but understanding and happy that you'll rearrange.

Remember...Choose to be calm. Choose to be positive. Choose to be happy!

Give in to your emotions

I'm going to completely contradict myself now. Remember you are a human. Beautiful, and vulnerable. That means that some days taking control of your emotions just isn't that easy. Some days I wake up feeling sad. I have no idea why. I do everything I can to turn it around. I exercise, meditate, repeat positive affirmations to myself, practise gratitude, eat chocolate and whatever I do, I cannot shift the dark cloud looming over my head. Some days I just have to give in to it and accept that for whatever reason, today is a sad day. And that's OK!

There is no such thing as a bad emotion. All emotions are a natural part of being a human. Some days these emotions will surface and, if you're anything like me, some days you'll have no idea why you feel the way you feel. It could be that you're carrying around the remnants of a dream you can't remember; it could be that your unconscious mind is processing something you're not aware of; it could be a hormonal change; it could be someone else's emotion you've picked up. Who knows?! When these days pop up, just try not to judge yourself for having these emotions. Vow to accept them for today and take extra good care of yourself. You'll probably feel much better after some rest and a good night's sleep.

Remember...tomorrow is a new day!

"*You can't calm the storm so stop trying. What you can do is calm yourself. The storm will pass.*"

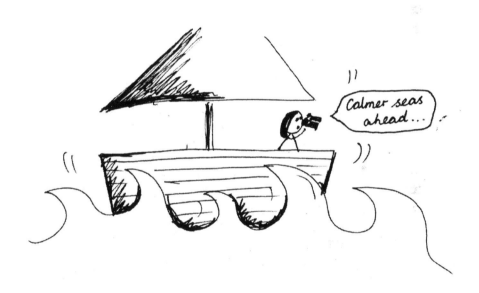

Improving your relationships

Getting in touch with your emotions can have a huge impact on the quality of your relationships. Regularly sharing how you feel with your partner/friends/parents, can save a lot of arguments! As females, our emotions are sometimes a little unpredictable and especially around a certain time of the month, we can become a tad more sensitive! In the past, if I was in a foul mood, I would have taken it out on my husband and not really thought anymore about it. I'm ashamed to admit it but when me and my husband first got together I was one of those people that would get a bag on (to translate for people not from Swadlincote, this means being in a mood/sulking) and then when asked what was wrong would inevitably answer, "NOTHING!" with a miffed face and sharp tone. I would probably have been grumpy with him for hours and spoil the whole day by not being able to communicate how I was feeling and being stuck in my emotions.

I now know that I'm able to do something to stop my mood affecting our relationship. I stop and ask myself, "Where is this emotion coming from? Has he actually done anything wrong? Could it be the way I am interpreting the situation? Could it be my insecurities being triggered?"

Sometimes I am annoyed with him just for walking through the door and he hasn't even had time to do anything wrong! Owning how you are feeling and communicating that to the other person is so important. It stops them from thinking that it's them in the wrong and then reacting defensively. I now might share with my husband, "I'm feeling annoyed with you but I'm not sure why yet. I'm sorry if I am snapping at you. Just bear with me while I figure out what is going on". My husband then knows he hasn't done anything wrong and that I'm taking responsibility for how I feel. Instead of carrying on the moodiness, I might just say, "I'm not feeling myself right now. Please can I have a hug?" At this point, instead of it erupting into an argument, we have a hug instead and that emotion dissolves. Just saying how you feel out loud to someone and having that physical touch and reassurance can make the black cloud drift away.

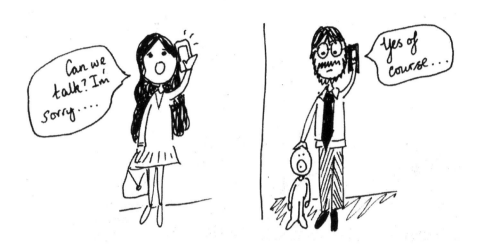

As I mentioned in the 'Challenge your thoughts' section, you need to take responsibility for your life and relationships. Once you become aware of your triggers, you can then choose how to respond. I have come to realise that I am very sensitive to rejection and any hint of this almost becomes evidence that my belief of 'I WILL BE REJECTED', will come true. I could quite easily create an argument about my husband talking to another woman or not giving me a kiss when he gets home – all of these things could be signs that I could be rejected. It wouldn't be fair of me to react negatively towards my husband every time these feelings are triggered, so I have to stop and question whether it is my stuff. Am I feeling this way because of my insecurities or is there actually something to be upset about? We are only human though and sometimes our emotions can get the better of us, making it very hard for us to stop and think rationally in the heat of the moment. However, it is never too late to communicate. If you feel you have overreacted to something. There is nothing stopping you from apologising afterwards and explaining, "I am sorry I reacted like that. I've thought about it and I think it was because I was feeling…" It's never too late to take control.

Remember…communication is definitely the key to dealing with difficult emotions.

Meditation

People often look at me like I'm a crazy hippy when I say that I meditate every day. Although, I think it has been become a more accepted practice in the last few years. I am by no means an expert but practising a simple daily meditation has really helped to calm my thoughts and my anxiety gremlins.

So, what is meditation? Meditation is basically concentration – learning to focus in the midst of our busy brains. We spoke earlier about being an observer to your thoughts. Well, that's basically it! I hear a lot of people say, "I can't sit still for long enough", "My brain's too busy, I can't switch off my thoughts". It's not about that – you can't stop thinking, the same way that you can't stop breathing or blinking. It just happens.

To meditate, take a few minutes to start with to sit/lie in a comfortable position, making sure you're not going to have any interruptions. Close your eyes. All you need to do is start focussing on your breathing. Breathing in. Breathing out. Noticing your belly rising and falling. Thoughts will start to creep into your head about what you're having for tea etc. It's natural to feel frustrated and want to give up, but gently push those thoughts away, tell yourself that you'll come back to them later and then refocus your attention onto your breath. Slowly in and out.

I would start off with 5 minutes a day and build the time up gradually. Meditating is a skill. You wouldn't go to the gym a couple of times and expect to have bulging muscles. It takes time, patience and practise. You need to work on building your meditation muscle.

So, how and why does meditation work?

Back in our caveman days, it was essential for survival that we were able to detect threats. Your body cannot determine the difference between a physical threat and a mental threat. Stress and anxiety are now our biggest threats. However, our brains are not designed to cope with the busyness that we experience in the modern day. When we were hunter-gatherers, we would have had periods of stressful activity when we were fighting off predators, hunting them and preparing them to eat, but then we might have days with very little activity where our minds and bodies would be able to recover. This is where we go wrong as modern humans. We don't allow ourselves the space and time to relax and recover.

Having constant high levels of mental and physical activity can lead to stress. When you're stressed, your body releases a hormone called cortisol. This then activates your sympathetic nervous system - your 'fight or flight' response. You may know this response well – tense shoulders, racing heart, sweating. However, too much cortisol can lead to all sorts of problems like inflammation in the body which is the cause of many health issues. In this state, your body's focus is to survive. It switches off any systems that it doesn't need, like your immune or digestive system. You might find that when you're stressed, you seem to pick up more colds or struggle to lose weight or suffer with IBS. This is why. Your body has gone into survival mode. This can also have an impact on the production of key hormones, such as testosterone, oestrogen or progesterone as your body is prioritising making cortisol. Therefore, if you're stressed and a woman, it's likely to affect your periods.

Meditation, mindfulness and deep breathing help to activate our parasympathetic nervous system. When our 'out-breath' is longer than our 'in-breath', messages are sent to our brain to say that we are not under threat and that our body is able to function as normal.

As I've said, meditation takes patience and practise, but there are many things you can do to help you to stay focussed on your breathing and stay present in the moment. Here are just a few suggestions:

If you count in your head while you're breathing, it will be harder for your brain to think about anything else. I usually use the **4, 7, 8** breathing technique...

*Breathe in through your nose (counting slowly to **4** in your head).*

*Hold your breath and count to **7** in your head.*

*Breathe out through your mouth (counting to **8** or more in your head, emptying your lungs).*

Or you might do something more simple like:

*Breathe in through your nose and, while doing so, say the following words in your head: "**In 2, 3, 4**..."*

*Breathe out through your mouth and, in your head, say, "**And out 2.....3......4......**"* This time you're counting more slowly to allow you to breathe out for longer.

Another breathing technique that you may find helpful is called **Box Breathing** or **Square Breathing**.

Start by closing your eyes and breathe in through your nose while counting slowly to four in your head.

Hold your breath while you slowly count to 4 in your head.

Slowly exhale through your mouth while counting to 4 in your head.

And then hold your breath while you slowly count to 4 in your head.

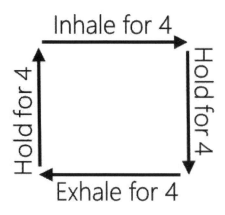

It can be helpful to imagine the box in your head as you breathe or follow the diagram with your finger so that you don't lose track of what you're doing.

Or I might repeat some of these affirmations to myself while I'm breathing to distract myself from intrusive thoughts...

I am present

I am calm

I am in control

Everything's working out

I am enough

I have enough

I can handle everything

If I'm finding it particularly difficult to calm my mind, I tend to put on a piece of instrumental music that I love that is around 10 minutes long. Towards the end, I might start thinking about the things that I am grateful for and the goals I am working towards. After 10 minutes, I feel refreshed and ready to start my day! I do this in the middle of the day too, if the boys are testing my patience or if I want to shake off a bad mood. There's no limit to how much you do it or when. For me, learning this has been life-changing.

There are lots of free apps, such as, 'Headspace' or 'Calm' that will guide you through a short meditation and help you learn how to do it. I often search for guided meditations or meditation music on YouTube and there's a wealth of videos on there to enjoy. You'll have to find the one that works for you. Sometimes the voice of the narrator can be quite distracting if you find their accent difficult on your ears - you'll need to find someone that fits. Don't let this put you off. Keep trying. You will feel the benefits.

Remember...you are not meditating for a reason other than to rest your mind. When your mind is quiet, the answers are clearer.

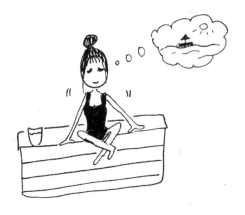

"The mind is like water, when it's turbulent, it's difficult to see. When it's calm, everything becomes clear."

Diaphragm breathing

So, you now have a little bit of an understanding as to what mindfulness and meditation are. They're both about concentrating on being in the moment and focussing on your breath. For you to get the full benefit from these though, you need to learn how to breathe. You might be thinking, "Doh! I think I know how to breathe! I've sort of been doing it my whole life!" Indeed you have but I doubt very much that you've been doing it correctly!

To fill your lungs to their capacity, you need to activate and strengthen the diaphragm muscle which lies at the base of your lungs. Here is a simple breathing exercise for you to incorporate into your meditation practise. This is good to practise lying down when you're learning how to do it as you'll be able to see more easily whether you are doing it right. Practising in the bath can also be a good place to start.

Lie flat on your back, with one hand on your chest and the other on your belly (just below your ribs). Imagine that you have a balloon in your belly and when you breathe in through your nose, imagine the balloon inflating and pushing out your belly. Your chest and shoulders should be still while you're doing this. All the movement should be coming from your belly. When you breathe out through your mouth, imagine the balloon deflating and feel your belly going in and getting smaller.

To simplify:

Breathe in – belly out

Breathe out – belly In

I not only practise diaphragm breathing while meditating, but also periodically throughout the day to keep me calm and slow my pace down. I breathe while I'm driving to pick the boys up from school. This helps me to mentally switch from 'counsellor/coach mode' to 'mum mode'. I breathe before I know I'm going to see a difficult family member to help prepare me to stay calm and be unaffected by their moods. I also may make an excuse to take myself to the bathroom and breathe whenever I am feeling overwhelmed/annoyed/frustrated in a situation. If you don't take anything else away from this book, then I would say that breathing in this way is the most simple and effective way to help control your emotions and calm your negative thinking.

Remember...the depth and speed of your breathing is what tells your brain you're not under any threat.

Grounding

Focussing on your breathing can be brilliant for anxiety. However, if you suffer with intense anxiety, panic attacks or flashbacks some people can find it helpful to shift their focus away from their body. When you're stuck in an anxious state, grounding techniques help to bring your attention back to reality and back to the here and now. Here are a few simple techniques that you might find helpful when your anxiety hits its peak:

1)   *54321*
Name out loud:

> 5 things you can see (shifting your attention to things further and further into the distance)

> 4 things you can hear (again, getting further and further into the distance)

> 3 things you can touch (get up and touch them)

> 2 things you can smell (or like the smell of)

> And take 1 deep breath.

2)   *Ask yourself questions and answer them out loud if you can...*
What is my full name?

What is my date of birth?

What is my address?

What is the date today?

Where am I?

Who is the Prime Minister?

3)   *Tapping the bone under your eye*

Tapping the bone under your eye socket with 2 fingers can feel uncomfortable and slightly painful. If you concentrate on this sensation, it can help to distract you from the difficult emotions you're feeling and help you to regain your focus in the present.

4) *Name everything you can see*

Winnie the Pooh did this in the Christopher Robin film! Literally name and describe everything you can see around you. Tree...road...red car...blue car...man walking dog...traffic lights...

5) *Alphabet Game*

Work your way through the alphabet finding an animal that begins with each letter. You could do this with girl's names/boys' names/Disney characters/Superheroes etc.

6) *Kind self-talk*

Tell yourself:

"I am safe"

"This will pass"

"I can get through this"

"I've been through worse than this and survived"

Remember...no emotion lasts forever. Stay with the anxiety, breathe through it, distract yourself and it will pass. The more you try and avoid the emotion the stronger it will become.

Safe place

Another way of calming your thoughts and creating inner peace is by closing your eyes and visualising a place that brings you happiness. It could be a beach that you went to as a child; walking through the woodlands in the springtime; having dinner with Mickey Mouse in Disneyland.

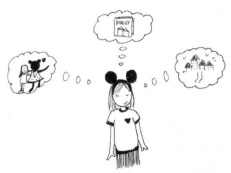

Wherever your special place is, use all your five senses to really imagine what it would be like there. Think about what you can hear. What can you see around you? Can you feel the sun beating down on your face? What can you smell? Is there anyone else there?

I tend to use this when I go to the dentist! I close my eyes, pretend I haven't got a drill in my mouth and imagine I'm lying on a beach with the waves rushing in and out in the distance, seagulls noisily flapping ahead and the warm, gentle breeze of summer brushing past my skin. It helps every time.

I wonder...where you would escape to in your mind?

Empty your head

As I said previously, I write in a journal every morning. I write down everything I'm grateful for; I set my intentions for the day (how I want to feel during the day) and what I'm going to do to care for myself that day. I have also started writing down anything that is playing on my mind and any niggling worries I have. This can help to lighten the load you're carrying around in your head. It can be helpful to write down your worries and then ceremonially get rid of them by screwing up the paper, ripping it up, burning it, sending it off down a stream and physically watch your worries float away. Writing them down isn't a magic cure to take the worries away, but any way that you can get them out of your head will help you to process them and eventually let go of them.

If writing isn't for you, I have known people to record themselves on their phone and then delete it or listen to it a week later to see if they're still worried about that thing. More often than not, that thing that was so significant wasn't as bad as they thought it would be, or it didn't even happen!

In whatever way you feel comfortable, empty your head of your worry gremlins. Talk to a friend or a counsellor. Take the anxiety's power away by talking about it in some way. Anxiety breeds on silence.

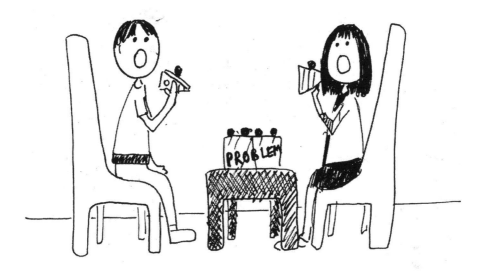

Remember...a problem shared is a problem halved.

Worry time

If you currently suffer or have suffered with anxiety, then you'll know how exhausting it is listening to the constant, negative intrusive thoughts that pop up at the most inconvenient time. They usually appear when you're meant to be listening to your children read, writing an important assignment or sitting in a meeting taking notes. To help combat this invasion and gain some control over these anxious thoughts, set yourself a time that is convenient for you to worry. If the thoughts are intruding then gently and without judgement, think to yourself, *"Isn't that interesting that I'm worrying about ...x... I'm going to choose not to think about that right now as I can't do anything about it but I will worry about that when I get home later".*

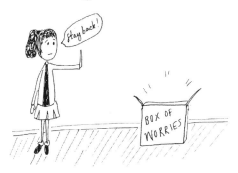

Set yourself a time, maybe between 7 and 7:15pm when the children are in bed, to think and worry about that thing until your heart's content! You're still allowing yourself to feel that emotion and have those thoughts, but by delaying them you are taking some control back. You might find that by the time it comes around to your worry time, you no longer need to worry.

Remember...be curious when listening to your anxious thoughts to maintain distance between you and them.

Monitoring your emotions

Technology has led to many of us being tied to our phones. There are so many downsides to having our phone with us constantly – it can prevent us from being present and mindful; it can get in the way of us connecting with others face to face; we compare ourselves to others on social media; we can easily spill our negative emotions to the world without considering the consequences.

However, there are some amazing apps and websites designed to improve wellness and mental health. There's a great free app called 'Woebot'. It checks in with you daily to see how you're feeling and depending on your response, it gives you advice or information that can help. We can get so completely sucked into life that our focus is very rarely on us and how we feel. These apps help you to stop and take a moment to reflect on how you're doing, providing reminders and tips on how to feel better. It can be useful to track your emotions, so that you can identify any patterns or triggers. Once you have this awareness, you can take appropriate steps to make changes.

Remember…the first step to controlling your thoughts and emotions is raising your awareness to them.

One year's time

When we're in the middle of an anxiety crisis, it can feel like the end of the world. It can be triggered by anything – your boss making a comment about your work; your friend cancelling a plan last minute or your mum making a remark about your parenting skills. You might stew on this for days. Just stop and take a deep breath and ask yourself, "Am I going to be bothered by this in a year's time?" or "Am I even going to remember that this happened in a year's time?" If the answer is 'no', allow yourself to be upset while you work through it, but set yourself a time limit so that you can move past it. If it's not going to have a big impact on your life, then it's probably not worth the time and energy that you would normally give to it.

Remember...you are in control of your emotions and your response.

"Inner peace begins the moment you choose not to allow another person or event to control your emotions."

PEMA CHONDRON

Step into the bubble

One of the first things I did while I was trying to get myself better was protect myself from negativity. I find that I absorb other people's emotions easily and take them on as my own. As a result of this, I came off Facebook as I didn't want to read anything negative; I stopped following certain friends on Instagram because their posts constantly triggered my insecurities about not being a good enough mum; I stopped listening to the radio, watching the news and reading newspapers as they made me feel sad and angry. People may think this is ignorant, but I say do whatever it takes to stay positive and mentally fit.

I fill my life with all things positive – music that I love, positive quotes, pictures and photos that make me smile. I really try to keep myself in my own little bubble of positivity! What could you remove from your life that has a negative impact on you?

I wonder...how could you create your own bubble of positivity?

Distance yourself from the mood hoovers

There are some people in life that thrive on drama. For whatever reason, they're not in a place where they want to seek help and instead spend their days moaning about what's going wrong in their lives. Do you know anyone like this?! When you have been around these people for any length of time, you can feel drained and like the energy has been sucked out of you. My friend refers to people as either being 'Drains' or 'Radiators' – I love this! 'Drains' drain you of your energy and 'Radiators' radiate positive energy.

As you start to take control of your mood and emotions, it may become apparent that you may need to start distancing yourself from negative people as your drama tolerance levels are likely to shift. I'm not saying that you need to cut people out of your life or fall out with anyone, just become aware of who you are choosing to spend your time with and whether they have a positive impact on your life.

The following model may help you to identify any relationships you have which aren't particularly good for you. This is a model of human relationships and interactions called 'The Drama Triangle', which was devised by Stephen Karpman. The model identifies the roles people can play in an unhealthy, conflictual relationship. The three roles are:

- **Victim** – the victim often interacts from a place of "Poor me". They feel helpless, hopeless, seem unable to make decisions, solve problems or take pleasure in life.
- **Rescuer** – the rescuer is known for saying, "Let me help you". Rescuers have a need to please people, a need to fix things, they feel guilty if they can't help, they focus their energies on others so that they don't have to focus on their own anxieties.

- **Persecutor** – the persecutor often interacts with, "It's all your fault". They are blaming, critical, angry, superior and rigid.

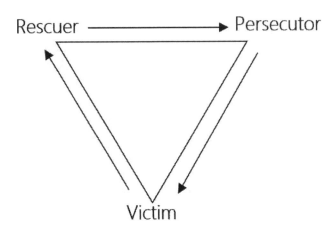

Karpman explains that as conflict arises, the people involved move around the triangle switching roles, but remain stuck in a destructive cycle. Take the following example...

Jennifer is married and has 4 children. She shares with her friend Amy that she is unhappy in her marriage and really struggling for money, to the point where she will struggle to do a foodshop this week and feed her children. This isn't the first time Jennifer has spoken about her money troubles. Jennifer often discloses things that are going wrong in her life, yet she rarely seems to take action to improve things - Jennifer is the Victim. Amy, feeling guilty that she is not in the same position as Jennifer, then acts as Rescuer to fix Jennifer's problems. She has bought Jennifer bags of food before, often gives her bags of clothes for the children and has spent a great deal of time listening to Jennifer's troubles. She feels the relationship is onesided as Jennifer never asks her how she is. After seeing her, Amy feels drained and often leaves feeling bad about herself.

A week later, Jennifer discloses to Amy that she had been on a shopping spree and had treated herself to expensive new shoes and a matching handbag. Amy feels confused. Jennifer has told her how much she is struggling financially and then spends money on things she doesn't need. Amy then moves to the Persecutor role as she becomes angry and critical of Jennifer's behaviour. Amy decides not to say anything this time. A few weeks later, Jennifer has the same problem and the cycle continues...that is until Amy decides to step out of it.

The way to step out of the drama is by stepping into 'The Winner's Triangle', devised by Transactional Analyst, Choy.

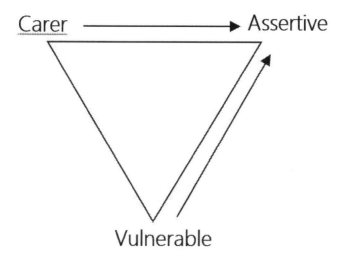

As you may notice, the labels on the triangle have changed slightly. The Victim has become the Vulnerable – they are still suffering and in pain but take action to take care of themselves. The Rescuer has become the Carer – they still have a concern for people and want to help but instead of jumping in to fix things, they listen, offer empathy and then put it back to the person by gently asking, "What are you going to do about it?" This then changes the label of Persecutor to Assertive. Instead of the individuals becoming upset with each other, this communication encourages the Rescuer to become more assertive and protect their boundaries; it also enables the Victim to start using their thinking to solve problems, encouraging them to become more assertive. The never-ending cycle is broken.

It doesn't always work this smoothly though. If you are a Rescuer, you might find that if you stop rescuing, the person will no longer need you and will replace you with someone else who can meet their needs. Sometimes, the Victim isn't ready to take responsibility and make changes. It feels safer and easier to stay stuck in the struggle and negativity. Equally, the Rescuers may not be ready to give up rescuing. Rescuing may provide a sense of purpose and a boost in self-esteem and without this behaviour, they may struggle to find their worth.

When I first became aware of this model, I realised that 90% of my relationships fit into the Drama Triangle! It was tough to make the shift towards relationships with more equality. I have lost touch with a fair few friends and family members because I was no longer prepared to be the Rescuer. Although this has been hard at times, I definitely don't feel emotionally exhausted and resentment like I used to. The people I have in my life now, even though it may not be many, are people I can trust, people that care about me as much as I care about them and people that don't just want a relationship with me because they 'need' me.

I wonder if any of this feels familiar to you? If so, which triangle do you find yourself on in your relationships? Which role do you tend to play?

So, you may have identified which relationships lean more towards the negative side, but like I said, you don't have to cut these people out of your life, it may just be a case of thinking about how you can manage them better.

It might be that you need to accept that spending an hour with your mum at any one time is the limit before the conversation turns sour and she starts to get on your nerves! It could be that inviting certain family members round at the same time causes you stress and that it might be better to arrange to see them separately. It might be that you need to steer conversations away from certain topics that in the past have caused defensiveness or conflict.

It can be helpful to write a list of the friends and family in your life. Circle the people that make you feel good, love you for you and don't need anything from you, and make a promise to yourself that you're going to put more time and effort into nurturing and strengthening these relationships. For the people that you haven't circled, you will need to decide how you're going to tackle these relationships – is it time to let them go or is it just a case of management?

Remember...your happiness is the most important thing that you have control over. Protect it with all of your might!

What are your strawberries?

At the start of my journey, when I was struggling with depression, I read a brilliant book called, 'The Endorphin Effect' by William Bloom. The book focusses on how you can reconnect with the beauty of life and find happiness again. It contains a perfect story to illustrate this...

One day a man was walking through a forest. He heard a rustling in the bushes behind him and out jumped a fierce and hungry lion. The man started to run through the forest and stopped as he came to the edge of the cliff. As the lion pounced out of the trees in front of him, he took a step back and the ground crumbled under his feet sending him over the edge. As he began to fall, he managed to grab hold of a root of a tree. As relief swept across his body, he looked up to see a tiny mouse gnawing away at the root. At that moment, the breeze brushed past his face bringing with it the sweet smell of strawberries. The man looked up and saw a strawberry plant with the juiciest, biggest, red strawberry he'd ever seen. The man reached with one hand and picked the strawberry...

The moral of the story is that no matter what life throws at you or what crisis you find yourself in, you can always find something that reminds you of the beauty of life. There are always positives if you look hard enough for them.

Finding those little moments are what make you truly happy. To find out what your strawberries are, make a list of all the things, big or small, that make you happy and then fill your days with as many of these are you can, as often as you can. Try to consider your five senses as you do this.

For example, some of my strawberries are:

Watching my boys sleep

'Hotel Chocolat' chocolate

Snuggly teddy bear blankets

The breeze on my face as I run

The smell of my vanilla cupcake Yankee Candle

Holding hands with my husband

Walking through the woods in the Spring

'You've been framed!'

Running with my puppy

'Miranda'

Monkeys

Disney

Dwayne 'The Rock' Johnson!

It can be useful to make yourself a little box that you can pull out in emergencies, when your mood is low. You could keep your box stocked with as many of your strawberries as you can - your favourite chocolate, candles, music, photos, favourite herbal teabags etc. It can be hard to remember what makes you happy when the cloud looms over head. It's good to be prepared – we all have bad days.

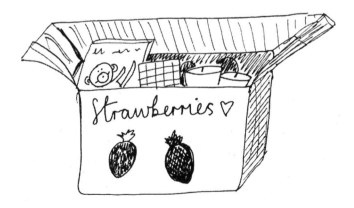

I wonder…what your strawberries are?

Make a mood board

To help start the day in a positive frame of mind, make a mood board. All you need is a cork notice board, some pins and fill it with all things positive. You might want to include: positive quotes; photos of loved ones; places you have been; places you would like to go; dream car; favourite animal – anything that makes you feel good when you look at it.

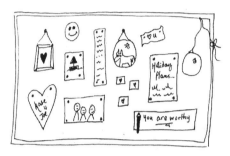

The act of finding the pictures, flicking through magazines, printing things off the internet, feels very therapeutic in itself. You know you're taking control of your happiness and doing something that's positive for you. I put my board at the side of my bed, so it was the first thing I saw when I woke up in a morning. I spent a few minutes every morning just looking at it and soaking up the positive feelings that it triggered.

I wonder...what you would put on your board?
What would you like to see first thing in a morning
that would help put you in a good mood?

Connect with friends

Earlier I mentioned the importance of stepping into a bubble of positivity, which is useful for protecting yourself against negative people and negative news stories etc. I want to make it clear that being in a bubble and isolating yourself are two different things. The latter not always being so helpful.

Sometimes when we're feeling low, we can distance ourselves from friends and family. We don't want to feel like a burden, we don't think we'd be very good company, or we haven't got the energy to face people, so we hide away. In my experience, this only makes the issue worse over time. You then begin to feel lonely and like no-one cares, which then confirms all the negative beliefs you originally had about yourself. You don't need to pretend. It's OK not to be OK. The people that love you want to be with you through your ups and your downs. Allow people in. Arrange to see a friend for a coffee, even if it's just for an hour. We humans are designed to connect with others. We need to feel that we belong.

Remember...no matter how rubbish you're feeling, make a commitment to yourself that you will contact one friend this week.

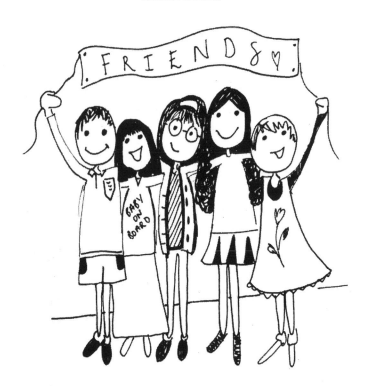

Four-minute rule

This is a great way to take control over your mood and have a huge positive impact on your relationships. If you're a working parent, then I'm sure you'll have experienced walking in from a stressful day at work and feeling annoyed that your wife/husband/children are immediately in your face! You may feel overwhelmed and get snappy with them because all you want to do is come in, sit down, have a coffee and unwind from your day. If you come home in a grump, it's not good for anyone involved. Especially you, because I imagine you'll then feel rubbish for not being able to leave your work stuff at work. It may help to be aware that the first four minutes of any interaction are the most important, as it this is what is remembered.

No matter how tired you are or how stressful your day has been, as you're driving back, ask yourself, *"How would the best mum/dad in the world greet their children? How would the best wife/husband in the world greet their loved one?"* You may need to muster up some energy and positivity, but the good thing is – you only need to keep it up for four minutes! You can do anything for 4 minutes! Once you've greeted them as super-mum/dad/wife/husband and everyone's happy, you can then sit down with your coffee and they'll be content to go off and carry on with their day.

Try this at bedtime too. How would the best mum/dad in the world read to their children at night? You will notice such a difference in your relationships, and you'll feel good for being in control of your emotions.

Remember...it's true what they say...'first impressions count!'

Woman's best friend

I never really got the whole dog thing! I didn't understand why people would allow their lives to be ruled by their furry friends and if I'm honest, over the years I've resented my family members' dogs, as I often felt that they were being put before me and my family. That was until I got my own dog. I completely fell in love and my life has not been the same since.

I have a beautiful, ginger cockapoo called Belle. You probably guessed that she was going to be named after a Disney character! They say that dogs look like their owners and you couldn't really get a better match. As a puppy her fur was exactly the same colour as my hair and she had a little white stripe on the left side of her head the same as me. She is my baby, my world and I love her nearly as much as my children! She brings absolute joy to all our lives.

Having a puppy was difficult, almost as difficult as having an actual baby and at times very frustrating, as all she wanted to do was bite me, but it's all been worth it. Seeing Belle's beautiful eyes, tilted head whenever I'm talking to her and wagging tail when I walk through the door instantly lifts my mood. She is my anti-depressant.

It is well documented that pets, especially dogs, can help improve your mood and overall mental health. When Belle is slightly older and doesn't get so excited as soon as someone walks through the door, then it is my intention to have her trained as a therapy dog for this reason. She would be a great asset to my private practice to help clients to feel relaxed in the sessions and help them to feel comfortable enough to open up. Stroking a dog can be incredibly therapeutic and help alleviate stress, anxiety and depression. Owning a dog can help to ease loneliness and improve fitness, as they make you go outside and you can't help but talk to other dog owners when your dog is adamant they want to say hello to every other four-legged creature you pass and sniff their bits!

I wonder...if you haven't got your own dog, do you have a family member or friend that has one you could borrow?

Move it, shake it!

Three years ago, I was lucky enough to go to Tony Robbins' 'Unleash the Power Within' Conference in London, which focussed on helping you to let go of your fears and insecurities and take steps towards creating the life that you want.

This was one of the key things that I took from the experience...your physiology (the way you move your body) is closely linked to your emotions. Picture yourself when you're feeling sad. Think about what your body language is like (probably closed, shoulders slumped, head low, no eye contact); how you talk (probably slowly, quietly, deeply); how you walk (again, probably slowly, feet dragging). On the other hand, think about what you look like and how you move when you're feeling happy, confident and motivated – the complete opposite, I imagine.

If you find yourself slipping into a bad mood, or if you're having an energy lull – GET UP AND MOVE! Change what you're doing with your body. Just standing up and stretching up to the ceiling while you take deep breaths in through your nose and out through your mouth, can help you to regain focus. Getting up in the morning and standing with your hands on your hips, legs apart, chest and head high (like a superhero) can help you to feel energised. You can't possibly feel the same level of sadness, annoyance, tiredness when you're breathing deeply and standing like Superman/Wonder Woman! Your physiology has a massive effect on the intensity of your emotions.

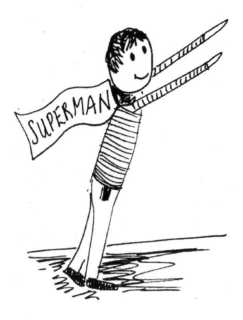

Remember...motion creates emotion.

Power moves

The way you move your body can also help to give you a boost of confidence or create a positive mindset. Before doing a presentation, going on a date, going to an interview, take a moment to get yourself in the right frame of mind. Whether you feel it or not, stand tall and confident. Shoulders back, head high and psych yourself up with some motivational self-talk.

Find something that you can do with your body to inject power, energy and motivation into you. You might punch the air, bang your chest, punch your open hand, shake your fists. Whatever feels right for you, do it with passion. Tell yourself, "F**king come on! Bring it on! I am f**king unstoppable! I am going to smash this!"

The more profanities you can use, the better, as it really helps to get your blood pumping! Richard Stephens, a psychologist at Keele University, found that swearing helps with empowerment but also pain management, and by inducing a spike in adrenaline, it can help increase strength and physical performance. I've done my power move so many times that I only need to tighten my fist slightly now and I get a rush of adrenaline and feel more powerful!

I wonder...what your power move would look like?

Energy...wiggle, wiggle, wiggle, wiggle!

Music can really have a positive impact on your mood. I have to have music on in the morning to get me going. It has to be the right sort of music though. I can't be doing with my husband's American teenage rock or whatever it is! It feels like my brain is being hammered by a pneumatic drill and it puts me in a foul mood.

I've recently remembered how much I love 90s dance music. It takes me straight back to my teenage years, when I was a weekly clubber with my home-made fluffy boots, glowsticks and cowboy hat! I'm also quite partial to a bit of early 2000s R&B!

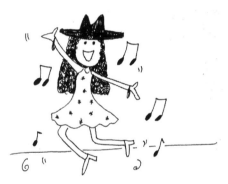

I put these songs on in the morning when I go for a run and race like the wind. It's a good job it's dark when I run because I can't always control myself and have been known to break out into a little lip-syncing, head-banging moment!

Are there certain songs that when you hear them make your body move uncontrollably?! Are there songs that instantly lift your mood? Why don't you make a playlist of all your favourite upbeat, energising songs and start your day with a dance party!

I wonder...what would be on your positive playlist?

Watch your language!

Your physiology can affect the intensity of the emotions you feel, but so can the language you use. How many times have you described being fuming or raging? As you are recounting a story, the words you use can intensify the emotion and help to build it up inside of you. When we're cross, we may add the odd choice word in there for effect as well. Try replacing high intensity words with less emotionally charged words. If you can add some humorous words in there, you'll certainly feel the difference as you're able to let go of the negative emotions that have a hold of you.

For example, try changing...

"I was raging" to "I felt a bit peeved"

"It was an absolute disaster" to "It was a tad disappointing"

"It was sooooo annoying" to "It was a bit of an inconvenience"

"I was terrified" to "I was a bit jittery, but excited"

"They were being a massive d**khead" to "They were being a bit of a unicorn"

(This cracks me up! Me and my husband use this as our code word for when our boys are being bothersome (notice how I didn't say annoying or p*ssing us off!). We will just randomly whisper the word 'unicorn' and have a little chuckle to ourselves!)

As I mentioned a moment ago, the language you use can also be used to intensify your emotions when you need an injection on energy or confidence. I have never been a big swearer. I wouldn't even say 'fart' never mind the other 'f' word! I used to think that swearing was a really negative, uncouth characteristic and I didn't understand the need for it. That was until I went to see Tony Robbins. I came back from that weekend, unrecognisable and swearing like a trooper! My eyes had become open to what my Welsh husband had been telling me for years, that to swear is to be passionate. It helps you to express yourself and feel energised about something. I still don't swear much in my everyday life, but it is certainly my go-to thing if I want to feel good. If I was feeling nervous about something, like going to a networking event or starting a new yoga class, I would be preparing myself with some positive affirmations and psyching myself up to taking on the new challenge.

I might be telling myself...

"I am f**king awesome!" (whilst clenching my fists and doing my power move!)

And my favourite (thanks to my husband!)...

"I am Claire f**king Reeves!"

If you are also someone who is usually very polite, try it! You'll feel so powerful as you drop the 'f' bombs!

> **Remember...if you want to feel more in control of your emotions, be aware of what is coming out of your mouth!**

Happy haven

I LOVE Disney! I used to be embarrassed about it and would worry that people would think I was weird or childish. Only a few years ago while I was in Disneyland Paris, I spotted a beautiful Ariel the Little Mermaid pen and notebook that I thought would be perfect for work, as having them in the office would remind me of our holiday. As I thought about the reactions of my colleagues, I reluctantly put them back on the shelf.

I now embrace it because it's part of me. It's part of my childhood. It's what I remember doing with my dad on a lazy Sunday afternoon before getting ready to go back to school. We'd cuddle up on the sofa and watch 'The Lion King' or 'Sword in the Stone' or one of the other classics. It reminds me of happy times and if I'm completely honest, I don't remember many of those. I remember arguments, tension, silence, as my mum and dad openly struggled with their marriage.

However, when I think of Disney, I think of love and happiness and that is what I have wanted to create in my own home, with my family. I now have a Disney-themed living room, with a beautiful collection of Disney ornaments that I'm very proud of. I also have positive quotes in every room and I have a random painting of a frog wearing glasses on my stairs just because it makes me smile every time I look at it!

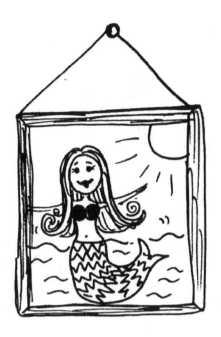

Remember…stop worrying about what other people think – it's not their house!

Cosy nook

I have found it really helpful to create a space where I can relax, reflect, read and meditate. If you have a spare room that you could dedicate to this then that would be amazing but unfortunately, we are not all that fortunate! All you need is a comfy cushion/chair/beanbag to sit on and anything else that will help to get you into the zone. I have some twinkly lights and a basket of lovely blankets that I can snuggle up in when I'm reading.

In your cosy nook, you might want to have:

- photos/pictures that you find relaxing and peaceful to look at
- incense or scented candles to help create a cosy atmosphere
- positive and inspiring books
- fairy lights
- your mood board filled with positive affirmations
- your daily gratitude journal
- a music player/headphones to play relaxing, meditation music

I wonder...what would you have in yours?

Hygge

Denmark is said to be one of the happiest countries on the planet and many people put it down to Hygge (pronounced Hooga). It's difficult to translate into English as we don't have a word for it! Basically, it's the feeling you get on a winter's day when you're cuddled up inside by the fire, wrapped in snuggly blankets, drinking hot chocolate. Hygge is a feeling – an atmosphere. It's about creating a cosy, safe, comfortable home which you share with your loved ones and where you're free to be yourself.

As I read more about it, I was pleased to know that I already lived this way! I spend my life in my knitted slipper socks; we all change into our pjs or comfies as soon as we get home; we love candles and lamps to create a cosy feeling.

So, what do you need to bring a bit of 'hygge' into your home?

Candles (and lots of them!)

Lamps/fairy lights

Hot drinks

Cake/pastries/rustic bread

Your favourite book

Good quality chocolate

Diffuser with lavender oils

A warm, woollen jumper

Slippers/slipper socks

Soft blankets

Cushions

Sheepskin rugs

Your favourite music

A bit of nature (plants, wooden furniture, wooden ornaments)

Board games

Cosy nook for reading/journaling/meditating

Gratitude journal

Movie nights

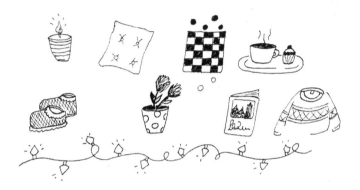

If you're aware of Maslow's 'Hierarchy of Needs' then it explains that in order for you to reach your full potential and self-actualise, you need to have your basic needs of safety, shelter, sleep and food met first. Introducing Hygge into your home and your life is bound to make you feel happier as your basic needs will be well and truly met!

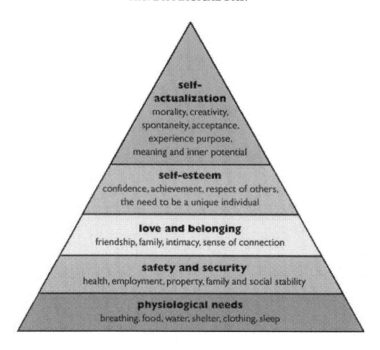

*Remember...it's the simple pleasures in
life that make all the difference!*

Healing with smells

If I am honest, it was only until recently that I recognised how powerful aromatherapy could be to help improve your mental health. I joined a new yoga studio and whenever I walked into the building, the lavender aroma massaged my senses, instantly making me feel lighter and like I could breathe. I wanted to find out what the smell was so that I could replicate it at home while I meditated, as I could feel how beneficial it could be to help me to feel calm and more relaxed. It also made me consider the aroma in my office, as I was aware that if my clients felt relaxed in the sessions, changes on an unconscious level were more like to be made. So, I bought an oil diffuser and began experimenting with different essential oils. I like to use a mixture - my favourite being lavender and peppermint or lavender and lemon. You can also apply certain aromatherapy oils to your skin on pulse points or buy them in a spray/mist to scent rooms or pillows.

So, how do they work?

Essential oils are highly concentrated plant extracts, which capture the aroma of the plant. They can be used as an alternative medicine to support psychological and physical well-being. Essential oils work by being absorbed by receptors in the nose connected with the olfactory system (part of the brain connected with smell). The inhaled oil molecules then activate the limbic system, which is linked to regulating our heart rate, blood pressure, emotions, breathing, memory and stress levels.

Here is a list of some of the common essential oils you might like to try and what they can be beneficial for:

Lavender – to relieve stress, improve sleep

Peppermint – to boost energy, aid digestion, improve memory

Sandalwood – to calm nerves and help focus

Orange – to decrease anxiety

Bergamot – to reduce stress, to improve mood

Chamomile – to improve relaxation, improve sleep

Tea tree – to boost immunity

Lemon – to improve mood, relieve headaches

I wonder...what smells help you to feel relaxed?

Dreeeeam....dream, dream, dream

Sigmund Freud was famous for quoting, 'Dreams are the royal road to the unconscious'. Your dreams are an incredibly powerful tool that can give you an insight into how you're feeling. Forget using dream books or Google for working out the meaning though. They are not always accurate. No one can interpret your dreams other than you because they are so personal.

Keep a notebook next to your bed and, as soon as you wake up jot down the main themes of your dream. Do this quickly so that you don't forget anything. You might be thinking, "Well, I don't dream!" – you do! Everyone dreams but not everyone remembers their dreams. Once you have jotted down your dream, go through each point and ask yourself, "What does this mean to me?"

For example, you might have had the following dream:

You were in an aeroplane. You were the pilot and you were struggling to control the plane. You realised that you were about to crash. You reached for your oxygen mask, but it was broken. You couldn't get it on, and you struggled to breathe. You started gasping for air. You felt so guilty that the people on the plane probably weren't going to survive. It was your fault.

Pick out the main themes of the dream:

Feeling out of control

Knowing that you were going to 'crash'

Things being broken

Struggling to breathe

Guilt and blame

Responsibility for other people's lives

You would then ask yourself if any of these things fit with how you might be feeling at the moment in your life. *Do you feel out of control in any area? Do you feel like things are too much? Like things are going to come crashing down? Do you feel suffocated in any area of your life? Is the weight of responsibility getting to you?*

You'll be surprised just how much your dreams reveal about how you feel at the moment. You might not have even recognised that you felt like that until you analyse the dream. Take this a step further though. Once you have an understanding of how you might be feeling, take action to give yourself what you need. For instance, if the above example applied then you might want to think about how you can start to take some control back. Do you need to lighten the load you feel you're carrying by delegating, asking for help?

Remember...to listen to the message of your dreams and take appropriate action.

Set your emotions free

There are consequences to not having an awareness of your emotions and not taking care of your mental health, as I have so painfully found out. Even though I have come along way, there is one thing I still struggle with and that is switching off and relaxing. I have at least 5 books on the go at any one time; I flit around starting but not finishing tasks around the house; I always have my laptop out doing *something*. I drive myself and my husband mad.

This behaviour is rooted in my limiting beliefs that if I am not doing *something* or achieving something then *I am not good enough*. This is something I have worked on in therapy for many years and had NLP coaching for and although there has been a big improvement in this area, I know it's still there from time to time.

Last year I was diagnosed with vestibular migraines which are migraines of the inner ear that cause dizziness and more so recently, horrible headaches. They started about 4 years ago when I had a bout of labyrinthitis which is an inner ear infection causing vertigo. That is quite simply one of the most horrendous things I've had. I couldn't drive, at times walk, lie down, be in the dark, be in bright light, watch TV without feeling as though my eyes were rolling in my head. Since then the dizziness has never gone away. I feel dizzy every day of my life. I feel as though I'm not quite attached to my body. This impacts so many areas of my life. I can't go on most rides with the boys, especially ones that involve virtual reality; I can't pick them up and swing them around like I used to; I can't watch 3D movies at the cinema; I can't watch certain moving things on TV or computer games; I find it hard to be a passenger in a car; I have had to cancel clients as I'm feeling so unsteady. I know people deal with far worse but for me this is hard. I feel limited which is something I am not used to. When the consultant explained that, in my case, the migraines were triggered by stress and anxiety, I laughed and completely rejected the idea. How could I still be stressed and anxious? I'd dealt with all that stuff. Anxiety was in the past! I was a changed woman! And, I was. I am.

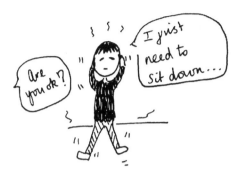

However, if I'm completely honest I'm still not great at being aware of what is going on for me. My focus, especially with the job I have, is usually about helping other people and being there for them. It wasn't until I had quite a difficult conversation with my husband where he made me see that anxiety is still very much present in my life and the impact it has on him and our family. I had been in complete denial! I felt I had lied to my clients when I had said that I no longer suffered with anxiety.

So how is this related to the dizziness? Well, the body and the unconscious mind are quite clever at making you stop and listen. I would suffer with migraines no matter what but they are usually made worse when I am stressed, anxious and after I've done something quite intense emotionally or physically. For example, if me and my husband have been away to Wales for the weekend to watch the rugby, I will probably have a migraine the next day. Whenever we've come back from Disneyland, I have suffered for a few days afterwards. Whenever, I have done something out of the ordinary or been upset...BAM!...there they are! It's become my body's way of slowing me down. When I am really dizzy, I literally cannot do anything. I don't think my body trusts that I will take care of myself and slow down, so it does it for me. So, since realising my physical condition was made worse by an emotional condition, I have taken many steps to improve my emotional self-care.

- I've changed the hours I see clients. I realised that doing three evenings a week was too much for me, so I work mostly school hours with one evening. I am working towards dropping evening work altogether by the end of the year.
- I used to see five to six clients a day and now I only see three to four which has really helped.
- I have joined a meditation and mindfulness class on a Sunday.
- I have joined a yoga class so that I am not just dabbling in it at home and I am socialising with other people (something I realised I wasn't really doing as I hadn't got anything left emotionally by the end of the week to have conversations with anyone).
- I have had hypnotherapy to really get rid of these stubborn limiting beliefs.
- I try not to cram too many things into one day and ask myself, "Do I really need to be doing this today or can it wait until tomorrow or the weekend?"
- I have started playing games on my boys' Nintendo Switch. I have been completely immersed in Zelda which has really helped me to relax and switch off.
- I keep an anxiety journal at the end of every day. I rate my dizziness and headaches on a scale of 1-10 and write down anything I've been anxious or stressed about.
- I have been arranging to see friends more so that I can't just fill my empty time with jobs and work.
- I have monthly massages to help me relax and release any tension I am carrying that might be contributing to my headaches.
- I have started asking for help more.
- If I've had a jam-packed weekend, I'll be mindful that I'll need to recover so I plan ahead and try not to

book as many clients in the next day.

Being self-employed really is a blessing, as I have the flexibility to fit my work in around my needs. I just need to be strict with myself to make sure that I am taking advantage of this flexibility and not falling back into old patterns of self-destruction.

Not listening to what you need and releasing the emotions you are feeling can lead to all sorts of medical problems. It is well-documented that unexpressed or unresolved emotional trauma and trapped emotions such as anger, can be the cause of chronic pain and conditions such as fibromyalgia. In my experience of working with hundreds of clients, once the emotional pain is dealt with, the physical symptoms they had also improve and in some cases disappear. Maybe the physical pain is the body's way of telling us that more emotional work needs to be done?

In best-selling author Louise Hay's book, 'You can heal your life', she attributes physical symptoms to emotional issues. Here are a few examples...

Pain in your head = self-criticism, fear

Pain in your neck = inflexibility in thinking, stubbornness

Pain in your throat = swallowed anger, inability to speak up for oneself

Pain in your upper back = lack of emotional support

Pain in lower back = money and financial issues

Pain in shoulders = carrying the burden of life

Pain in hips = fear of moving into the future, making decisions or of a change

Pain in knees = giving yourself too much credit, having an in-

flated ego, inability to bend

If you would like to find out more, there are some brilliant books out there, such as, 'The Body Remembers: The Psychophysiology of Trauma and Trauma Treatment', by Babette Rothschild and 'The Body Keeps the Score: Brain, Mind and Body in the Healing of Trauma', by Bessel van der Kolk.

A great way of releasing some of this pain and discomfort is raising your awareness to how you feel when the pain is bad. First of all rate your pain out of 10 and then repeat to yourself, out loud if possible, "I am feeling..." and fill in the blank. You keep repeating this until the pain has decreased to a 1 or 2 or gone completely. It might be something like this...

I am feeling sad.

I am feeling sad.

I am feeling frustrated.

I am feeling angry.

I am feeling sad.

I am feeling overwhelmed.

It doesn't matter if you keep repeating the same emotion over again. Listen to your unconscious mind and whatever you feel you need to say, let it come out. By doing this, you are demonstrating to your mind and body that you are listening and that you are willing to release these emotions. This has really helped with my dizziness. I just used to push through it before but now I stop, reflect and release.

I am a Certified Master Practitioner in Timeline Therapy. This is an amazing therapeutic process, which has evolved from hypnosis and NLP, to help with just this. It involves using visualisation to revisit past events to release the negative emotions of anger, sadness, fear, hurt and guilt and a limiting belief. It is like having a detox for your mind to help you to shift any emotional baggage that you've been carrying. If you want to find out more about this then you are welcome to contact me directly or visit www.timelinetherapy.com.

Remember...body and mind are deeply connected – you need to take care of both.

In summary...

Your emotions are designed to provide you with messages. It is really important that you take time every day to check in with your emotions and listen to the messages your mind and body are sending. As I've just said, your body is very good at communicating with you physically if you are not paying attention to your emotions and taking care of them. Your emotions can be affected positively or negatively, by the people you surround yourself with, the food you put in your body, your hormones, your language, your posture, your sleep. It is worth regularly giving yourself a little mental MOT and reflecting on all the above.

Asking yourself questions like...

"How do I feel about my relationships at the moment?"

"Is there a certain person that brings my mood down when I've spent time with them?"

"Is there is a certain food/drink that triggers my anxiety?"

"How is my sleep at the moment?"

If you've tried all of the things in the book and your mood is still low or your emotions feel quite erratic then it may be worth a trip to the GP to get further advise, as medical conditions such as an overactive thyroid can have symptoms that can affect your mental health.

COMPASSION AND CONFIDENCE

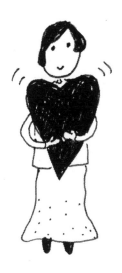

*"Having compassion for yourself means you honour
and accept your imperfections and humanness."*

Compassion And Confidence

If you've suffered with any sort of mental health illness, then you may have felt at times that someone else had taken over your brain. When I suffered with post-natal depression, I felt I had lost all sense of who I was - I had absolutely no idea what I liked and didn't like anymore. I felt completely flat and numb inside. When I started my journey, one of the things I had to do was rediscover ME. I learnt to appreciate that I wasn't perfect, which is something I had strived to be all my life, but that I was perfect because of my imperfections – they were what made me, ME.

Next are some of the things that I've done over the last few years to find myself and be truly happy with who I am. I hope you find them as helpful as I did. So far, the book has covered how you can change your thinking and emotions to feel better about yourself and the world around you. This chapter is more about your behaviour and the things you can *do*. It's OK to think nice things about yourself, but if you don't look after your emotional or physical needs, then the changes will probably not be long lasting.

Remember...it takes changes in your
thinking and actions to make progress.

I love myself

I read an amazing book called, 'Love yourself like your life depended on it', by Kamal Ravikant. It talks about making a commitment to love yourself. To not just accept who you are or like yourself, but truly love yourself. You might be thinking that's easier said than done, especially if you've spent a whole lifetime criticising yourself and putting others first. I imagine the practise that I'm going to share with you may feel uncomfortable, big-headed, self-righteous even, but if you can't commit to loving yourself, then you can't expect anyone else to do so. You probably won't believe it to start with, but you need to repeat these words to yourself a thousand times a day – when you're brushing your teeth, when you're waiting for the bus, when you're waiting for the kettle to boil. 'I LOVE MYSELF! I LOVE MYSELF! I LOVE MYSELF!'

Standing in front of the mirror and saying it can feel very powerful. This doesn't mean you think you're better than other people. It doesn't mean that you don't love your family and friends. It just means that you are showing yourself the kindness you might not have received in life, but that you deserve. The more you repeat this, the more it will become part of your unconscious thinking. Remember, the way you think also shapes your behaviour. So, the more you think you love yourself, the more you'll treat yourself like you love yourself. The more you love yourself, the more the world will love you.

To help you to say 'no' to people and situations that do not feel right for you, Ravikant says you should ask yourself, "If I loved myself, would I let myself experience this?" In my journal, I ask myself, "What can I do today to show that I love myself?", to focus my attention on looking after myself as well as everyone else.

**I wonder...how your life would change
if you loved yourself more?**

Build a compassionate image

If you find it difficult to show yourself love and kindness then the following exercise, based on the work by Paul Gilbert in his book, 'The Compassionate Mind', can be really helpful. It is designed to help you to build an image of a person/object/thing that can provide you with nurture, care and compassion.

Start by finding a comfortable place where you will not be interrupted. Close your eyes and with a half-smile on your face, concentrate on breathing in and breathing out. Go with the natural rhythm of the breath. Allow images to come into your mind of your compassionate person/object and ask yourself:

- Would you want your image to be male or female?
- Young or old?
- Would it be a person, animal, object, place?
- What would they look like?
- Are there any sounds that are important?
- If it's a person, is it someone you know? Have known?
- What qualities do they have? Wisdom? Strength? Warmth?
- Are there any colours associated with it? Imagine that compassionate colour surrounding you, flowing through you.
- How would they show you care? What would they say? Do?

Visualise this image sending you love and kindness. When you have mastered this and feel comfortable accepting compassion from your image, I wonder if you could change the image so that you are the compassionate person? Imagine yourself having all the qualities above. Imagine yourself being strong, wise and warm. Imagine how you would speak to yourself and treat yourself without blame or judgement. Imagine the 'compassionate you' reaching out and giving you what you need. Holding your hands in theirs. Embracing you. Stroking your hair. Kissing your forehead. Looking at you with kind eyes. Doing whatever it is that makes you feel cared for.

Remember throughout, breathe steadily and allow your body to relax into this. If you find visualising the image difficult, just concentrate on your breathing and with kind acceptance, remind yourself that it is OK. You are showing yourself compassion just by giving yourself this space to relax.

You may have a memory that you can work with to give you compassion. Can you think back to a time when someone in your life has been kind to you? Focus on the words they said, their tone of voice, and their body language. What was happening in the image? Imagine revisiting that experience where you felt totally loved, safe and accepted. Allow a feeling of gratitude to build inside you for that experience and have a knowing that you can visit it anytime you need a little boost in self-care.

Another exercise for you to try...

Imagine that with every breath, you are breathing in a colour that you find calming, warm and that you associate with compassion. For your out breath, breathe out a colour that represents self-doubt, blame, judgement.

Breathe in compassion.

Breathe out judgment.

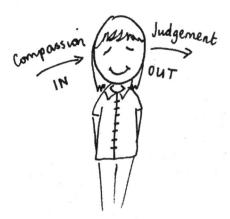

Imagine the compassionate colour expanding within your body, filling your chest, surrounding your heart. You can even imagine sending out that compassionate colour to the people who you love.

Whenever you are struggling, just close your eyes and bring your compassionate image to mind and allow yourself to soak up the love and kindness that you so need.

Remember...compassion will always be there with you. You can tap into this resource when you need it just by closing your eyes.

Love the mini-you

As adults, with our many responsibilities, deadlines and limiting beliefs, it can be quite hard to put ourselves first. Some of us have learned that we're only good enough if we are doing things for others. Some of us, for whatever reason, have learned that we're not important. Some of us, have learned that we're not worthy of love and care. We have these beliefs because our needs weren't fully met as a child. Now this doesn't mean that our parents didn't love us, or that they neglected us in anyway, it just means that there were times when we needed more than was on offer. If you are finding it hard to take care of yourself in the here and now, it can be helpful to start by bringing the 'little you' to mind. This is called Inner Child work. As adults, we are just bigger versions of the child we used to be. We probably have all the same insecurities and worries, we're just bigger. We all want to be loved. We all want to be accepted. We're just in a bigger outer shell.

Find a photograph of you, or if you don't have a photograph, just close your eyes and visualise you as a toddler. Think about what you liked at that age, what life was like for you, who was important to you and more importantly, was there anything you needed back then that you didn't have? Was there anything in particular you needed to hear or feel? Hold the photograph in your hand and imagine that if that little person was in front of you now, what would you say to them? What would bring them comfort? Encouragement? Love? Acceptance? Would you give them a hug? Would you tell them how special they are? *What did you need??* It can feel slightly easier to offer care and empathy to an innocent child than it can to our adult selves. Repeat this with photographs of you throughout the different ages and notice where you have the most connection. Notice where the pain is and where you were lacking the most.

For me, it was my teenage years when my mum and dad were getting divorced. When I look at photographs of me around the age of 15/16, I can see the pain behind my smile. I can easily take myself back there and feel what I felt. I felt my needs weren't important. I felt I wasn't listened to. I felt it was my job to look after everyone and that I couldn't rely on others to look after me. Unfortunately, I've carried this into my adult years and have had to work hard to undo this damage through my own therapy and self-development work. If I'm honest, I haven't completely shifted this and that is why I still find it hard to relax and put my needs first. It's a work in progress!

A lovely, but somewhat difficult way of communicating with your inner child is writing them a letter. Writing them a letter, containing all the things you needed to hear back then. What would you say to them to help them to get through that difficult time? What advice would you give them about life, love, relationships? How would you let them know they are important, worthy of love and good enough?

Along with my affirmations in my bathroom, I also have a small photograph of me as a child. This acts as a reminder to care for myself; to care for that innocent, sweet, little girl. To recognise that I am still her and that I need love too.

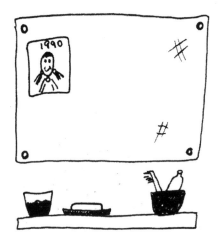

Remember...we are all just innocent children that want to be loved. Show yourself compassion and heal the pain from the past.

Fill up your self-love tank

For me, this has been the hardest one to crack and if I'm being completely honest, I'm still rubbish at this! As I mentioned in the previous section, I have always found it hard to relax. I feel guilty, lazy even, and think I should be doing 'something'. When I finally allow myself time to relax, I then seem to develop decision paralysis! There are then too many things I want to do that I don't know where to start and I end up getting quite stressed about relaxing! It can be helpful to write a list of all the things you like to do, so that you can whip it out if you're struggling to work out what you need at that moment. You could have things like run a bath, read a book, go for a walk, ring a friend. I know these may seem like simple suggestions, but I know that when I'm stressed, I forget the basics.

You may be thinking that you haven't got time for self-care. I used to say the same..."I've got the ironing to do", "I need to make the dinner", "I've got to finish my uni assignment", "I need to make a Children in Need costume for the boys", "I've got to do the food shopping" etc. I'm not saying that you don't have a lot to do. Trust me, I get it. However, life is about living and being happy – it can't all be about work and looking after others. This is your life too! There has got to be a balance.

One way to make sure you relax and spend some time caring for yourself is by making a promise to yourself to spend 10 minutes every day doing something just for you. It can be as simple as actually sitting down and drinking a whole cup of tea! Whatever you do - do these things mindfully – be present. Know that you're doing it for you because you deserve the same love and care as you give everyone else. You cannot care for others if you're running on an empty tank.

This is my list...

Paint my nails

Put on a face mask

Read a book

Buy a chocolate bar from the shop and enjoy every second of eating it!

Do some colouring/sketching

Have a bath with candles

Have an Ovaltine at the end of the day

Catch up on 'The Great British Bake Off'

I wonder....what could you do? Fill up your love tank and then share the love!

Schedule in your downtime

I find doing nothing really stressful. I never stop. I cram as much as I possibly can into a day without having much thought about the impact it could have on me. This is at its worst when I am feeling run down. The more exhausted and run down I am, the more I do. It drives my husband bonkers! A perfect example would be me telling my husband that I need a break and I'm struggling mentally and then inform him that I'd spent all day looking at other university courses to do! To me it makes perfect sense, it is only when I'm feeling back on form that I think, "Why on earth was I looking at going back to uni when I have enough to do!" It almost, at times, feels like a form of self-harm. In my mind, if I'm not achieving then I'm not existing. I suppose this all comes back to that 'not good enough' belief. I have been known in the past to completely freak out on a Saturday morning if we've got a whole weekend with nothing to do. My brain cannot handle the empty space. My husband doesn't get it as he can easily switch off and fill his days with the things he enjoys.

I must admit this need to always be on the go has really shifted since doing my NLP and hypnosis training. I do feel like I have let go of this and my self-care has improved dramatically. On the days I do find this hard though I will make myself a plan for the day so that the empty time feels more manageable.

A timetable of relaxing activities – which might look something like this:

5:30-6am – run

6:30-7am – meditate and do journal

7-7:30am – have breakfast and drink tea

8-9am – read my book in the bath

9-10am – put on my make-up and paint my nails

10-12pm – play board games with the boys

12-1pm – make lunch, eat and watch TV

1-2:30pm – walk Belle round the lake

2:30-4:30pm – visit my mum

4:30-5:30pm – make tea and eat

5:30-7:30pm – watch a family movie

7:30 – 8pm – put the boys to bed

8-9pm – read my book and listen to music

9-9:30pm – get ready for bed

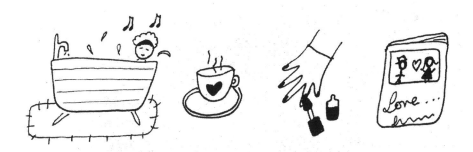

This might not work for everyone but for me, breaking the day down like this can make it feel less overwhelming. I am relaxing but tricking my brain into thinking that I am achieving at the same time! Planning the day can also help me to see that I'll be spending quality time with the boys and then don't feel guilty for the 'me' time throughout the day.

Remember...rest is just as important as work.

"Almost everything will work again if you unplug it for a few minutes... including you."

ANNE LAMOTT

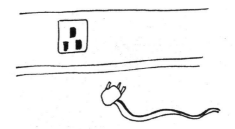

Recharge your batteries

I am a HSP. A Highly Sensitive Person. Psychologist Elaine Aron coined the term in the 1990s to describe people with a personality trait that involves an increased sensitivity of the central nervous system. HSPs are easily overstimulated as they process external stimuli on a cognitively deeper level than most other people. I am not alone though - HSPs make up about 15-20% of the population and can have the following characteristics:

- A heightened response to stimuli such as pain, caffeine
- Easily overwhelmed by bright lights, strong smells, loud noises, such as sirens, course fabrics
- Easily startled
- Conscientious
- Easily stressed when there is a lot to do in a short amount of time
- Avoidance of violence on TV shows/movies
- Sensitive to the change in people's moods
- Overly empathic and affected by other people's emotions
- Overly nervous in situations where they are being observed
- The need to withdraw after a busy day
- Easily moved by the arts
- Told as a child that they were 'too shy' or 'too sensitive'

When I read Elaine Aron's book, 'The Highly Sensitive Person', I had finally found the answers to explain everything about me. Why I cried watching random adverts on TV. Why I could tell the mood of my manager just from the sound of her footsteps. Why I hated presentations so much. Why I became hangry (angry when hungry). Why I felt my head was going to explode when the TV was a notch too loud. Why I fell sleep instantly in highly emotional situations.

I know some people disagree with giving people labels but for me this label changed everything. I felt normal and if anything, felt I could embrace these things about me instead of being frustrated with myself all the time. Elaine describes this sensitivity like having a superpower. We can see, feel and sense things that most other people can't. I now accept these quirks as part of me. They are my superpower.

I realised that just by being alive and functioning on a day to day basis, my nervous system was already working on over-time. No wonder I constantly felt frazzled and needed so much sleep. I am now a lot more aware of my triggers if there has been a change in my mood. If I find that I am snappy for no reason, I look at what is going on around me and usually it is because I'm being over-stimulated! Being in the car is the worst – my husband's put on a song by some weird American band that grates on my brain, the music is too loud, I'm having to shout to be heard over the music, the fan is making a noise, it's blowing cold air at me (I don't function well when I'm cold), the boys are laughing and making noise in the back of the car, the car is moving which sets off my dizziness. Sometimes I could scream! It has made me realise how difficult I can be to live with at times, but my husband has learned what my triggers are and can usually see what I need first. If I am hungry and tired, then I am a nightmare! He will casually ask, "Do you need a biscuit?!" As much as I usually reject that remark, he's normally right, as soon as I've eaten, the angry, black fog lifts and I am back to normal. It really is a Jekyll and Hyde situation.

Having this new knowledge and awareness has really helped me to take my self-care up another notch. I realised that I needed to give myself more time to recover from daily stressors. Now, I try not to squeeze too many things into one day. I look at achieving one thing a day on top of the normal, every-day jobs. I make a list at the beginning of the week of things that need to be done like, make a dentist appointment, ring SKY to query my bill, take the parcel back to Next etc. I pick one job to do every day, instead of trying to do everything all at once. If I can feel myself getting sucked back into the need to be 'doing things', I now ask myself, "Does this really need to be done today?" Most of the time it can wait.

I also give myself little rewards for doing jobs. An example is a while ago, both of the cars were embarrassingly filthy - inside and out. I didn't want to waste money by taking them to a car-wash, so decided it was a good idea to do them myself. It was not a good idea to do it on a day when it was -1 degrees! I was knackered afterwards and could not feel my fingers, it was that cold. Normally, I would have come in and got straight on with the next job. But instead, realising that I had worked hard for nearly 2 hours, I needed time to rest. I made myself a lovely mug of hot chocolate, ran a hot bath and read my book for the next hour. I felt proud that I'd achieved something but felt prouder that I was taking care of myself. If you don't put yourself first, or reward yourself, then why would anyone else?

Remember...being highly sensitive is a superpower!
It does however drain your emotional energy,
so good quality self-care is essential.

Spread the love like Robin Hood

Being kind to others for no reason is a really good way of showing love to yourself. It fills you with a warm, fuzzy glow and makes you feel good about yourself. It helps you to connect with others, which is what we humans are designed to do. Try setting yourself a goal of doing a random act of kindness every day for a week (or a month if you really want to go for it!) and see how great you feel. One of my favourite episodes of 'Friends' is where Phoebe is going around trying to do nice things for people without feeling good herself. It's not possible! Spread the love!

Remember that if you have people in your life who are particularly difficult and unkind then it's those people who usually need kindness more than others. This can really help to heal these relationships as it's usually unkind people who are filled with the most sadness and insecurities. Even if they are not receptive to your thoughtfulness - *kill 'em with kindness anyway*, you'll still feel great!!

Remember...hurt people, hurt people.

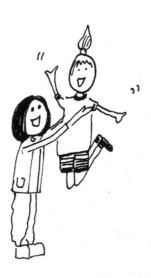

"We rise by lifting others."

ROBERT INGERSALL

Touch therapy

Physical touch is incredibly important. We need this to feel connected. From the moment we are born, physical touch is an essential part of forming bonds with our caregivers. We need it to survive. Studies have shown that babies deprived of physical touch, do not develop physically and mentally, at the normal rate and can even die.

Touch helps to lower the heart rate and reduce our cortisol levels, allowing us to move from our fight or flight state to our rest and digest state. If I find myself snapping at my husband, instead of allowing my mood to cause an argument, I will ask him for a hug, apologise for snapping and instantly my mood is lifted. Whatever it was that I was upset about disappears. Hugs and touch promote the release of serotonin and oxytocin, the body's natural anti-depressants.

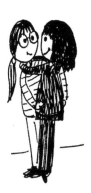

Even a gentle touch on the shoulder or back can lift your mood, as we have particularly sensitive receptors in this part of our body. This is why having a massage is helpful for relieving stress. It helps to release tension, ease pain but also can help improve your mental health.

I understand that not everyone likes to be touched and we

must respect that. If you are a tactile person though and you know it makes you feel better to have a hug, then do it more. Book yourself in for that massage. Play fight with your children. Hold your partner's hand. Lightly touch a friend on the shoulder when saying thank you. Let the positivity flow.

Remember...to get your quota of touch in as many ways as you can and get connecting again!

Be a child again

As we get older, we can lose who we are and stop having fun. As I've said before, there needs to be a balance in your life – work, family, exercise and PLAY! Growing up, I spent hours and hours drawing Disney characters and colouring. I loved anything arty. I loved singing and would spend hours recording the top 40 on Radio 1 on a Sunday night. I would write down the words to my favourite songs and sing them until I knew them off by heart. I loved dancing and even in my late teens (more like 20s!), I would watch music videos over and over again, to learn the dance routine. Me and my best friend would perform the routine in my mum's tiny kitchen – we thought we were the bomb! I loved being outside on my bike, roller boots, playing football, doing cartwheels in the field behind our house.

I felt embarrassed when I started drawing Disney characters again, but I just thought, so what?! What difference does it matter what other people think? Ariel the Little Mermaid was my favourite as a little girl. She was the first character I'd seen on TV with red hair; she was beautiful; she was a princess and she could sing – what was there not to love? I wanted to be her. She was proof that red hair didn't have to be an unattractive feature. Throughout my own journey, I have worked hard on self-acceptance. As part of this I decided to have a mermaid tattoo down my thigh as a reminder of who I am. I also chose to have it on a part of my body that I was self-conscious of, to help me to accept my body.

I now make sure that music and singing are a part of my days. There is nothing better than doing the ironing or being stuck in traffic and singing the entire Frozen soundtrack at the top of my lungs! That's my therapy!

I absolutely love 'Miranda' for this reason – she doesn't take herself or life seriously at all and embraces her somewhat child-like qualities. This is what makes her such a loveable character because she has the courage to be herself. She is so right – galloping is the future of happiness!

I wonder what you liked to do as a child? Write a list of all these things and incorporate them into your life. This is who you are.

***Remember...do what makes you happy
and embrace who you are!***

Get your creative juices flowing

Is there something you've always wanted to try? Belly dancing? Playing the saxophone? Pottery? Tapping into your creative energy can be a brilliant way to improve how you feel. Doing something simple and creative, like an adult colouring book, can have many benefits – it can help improve your levels of concentration; help you to relax; calm your thoughts; give you the brain space to work through problems and provide you with a sense of pride and achievement when you've completed it. When you've succeeded, your brain is flooded with dopamine, which is the chemical that makes you feel happy, and who wouldn't want to feel happier? Being creative and experimenting with new ways of doing things can help you to become more flexible in your thinking. This can help with problem solving in your everyday life and help to lower anxiety. Being creative can also help you to work through difficult emotions. You may find that creating a piece of art based on your experiences and emotions can help you to process and release them.

Just remember that there should be absolutely no pressure from others or yourself whilst doing your creative activities. **This is just for you.** It doesn't matter how good you are at it. Do it because you enjoy it and because it makes you feel good. I absolutely love watercolour painting. I find it incredibly relaxing and rewarding. If it ever starts to feel like a chore or I become frustrated, then I walk away and go back to it when I'm able to enjoy it again. You might find that you have a talent you didn't know you had! Just be prepared that if you find you are good at something, people will want to enjoy your talents too and may ask you to do things for them. Remember what I said about politely saying 'No'. If you want to do things for others, then great, but remember the idea of this is that it's something to help YOU.

I wonder...what will you try first?

Celebrate everything!

Most people I speak to describe living with a feeling of pressure. Pressure to have everything done and be on top of things, despite working full time, having children and having a house to run. Most of the pressure we feel though is pressure we put on ourselves. When you have so many responsibilities, it is inevitable that at some time, some of these things are going to suffer. You are not superhuman. Just think, if your children are clean and healthy, does it really matter if you haven't listened to them read every day this week? What long term impact is that really going to have? If you've met your deadlines at work, does it really matter if you reply to the rest of your emails in the morning? If you have clothes to wear for the week, does it really matter if you still have an overflowing ironing basket?

Most of the jobs that you do can wait. If you are honest with yourself, life isn't going to fall apart if you stop doing half of the things you say you have to do. Other than breathe, there's literally nothing that you HAVE to do in a day. Listen out for the words you use. How many times a day do you say, "I need to", "I've got to", "I should"? You don't NEED to do anything.

Try writing yourself a job list and cross off everything that can wait or that you don't actually want to do. Choose 3 things that you are going to aim to get done that day.

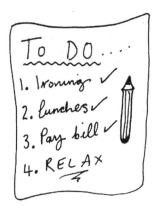

When we are feeling overwhelmed by the amount of jobs we have to do, it can be quite easy to focus on all the things we haven't managed to do. But I don't think we realise how much we have actually achieved in one day. At the end of the day, get into the habit of writing a list of all the things you've achieved and things you can be proud of. It can be as small as brushing your teeth; getting the children's lunches ready; handling a tricky situation at work. No matter how small, at the end of each day tell yourself...'I AM FREAKIN' AWESOME!!' and celebrate all that you have achieved. I use the 'Daily Greatness Journal' which has questions like this to help with daily reflection.

Remember...there will always be more to do. Do the minimum to get you through and then spend the rest of the time caring for yourself and your family and having fun!

Say "NO!"

When you don't value yourself, you tend to put everyone else's needs before your own. People then take advantage of this and you may find yourself doing things you really don't want to do - lending people money that you don't really have and generally doing things to please them. If you find yourself doing things because of the following: fear, obligation or guilt (or F.O.G. for short), then please question whether this is a healthy relationship. These will never feature in a positive, healthy relationship.

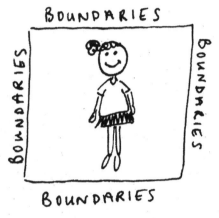

Saying 'no' and putting boundaries in place is the most powerful thing that you can do for yourself. You're saying to yourself, "I matter too". If you're not used to doing this, it can feel uncomfortable to start with and you may experience a wave of guilt afterwards, but please push through this. Try saying 'no' to small things first.

The hardest thing I've done is putting boundaries in with my mum. When my boys were babies, my mum used to call round to my house on her way to work to see them. At times it was a big help having an extra pair of hands. As the boys got older and as I went back to work, her calling round became less helpful. I'd be busy getting the boys ready, myself ready, packing bags for the day – anyone with children knows what mornings can be like. My mum would call in for 10 minutes, innocently asking me questions and want a conversation with me and the boys, but they obviously take after me because we're not great communicators in the morning. It takes me a long time to wake up and have the ability to form words! I would find myself snapping at my mum because I had a million and one other things to do and a very thin patience. Then I'd spend the rest of the day feeling like a terrible person. I finally plucked up the courage to suggest that it might be better if she came after work. My mum didn't get the gentle suggestion and proceeded to come around, always with a reason as to why it needed to be at that time. This continued for months. Every time the doorbell rang loudly at 7:00am, I thought my head was going to explode. I felt misunderstood and not listened to.

In the end, I felt I had to be a bit more assertive in the delivery of my message. I made it clear that it wasn't that I didn't want to see her, it just wasn't a great time and I didn't want to upset her by being snappy. Let's just say my mum was very upset and took it very personally! The upset eventually faded and we got things back on track. My mum very, rarely comes around at that time now and in fact she often rings or texts to see if I'm in before popping round, which I really appreciate. As I am writing this, I can feel the guilt washing over me! The thought of upsetting anyone, especially my mum, absolutely crushes me to the point where I feel I can't breathe. I love my mum to bits but sometimes you have to do what's right for you. Sometimes that means risking upsetting people but remember...you are not in control of people's emotions, only your own.

Another thing I started doing when I was trying to put boundaries in place and put my needs first was not answering the phone at an inconvenient time. I know it might sound awful but if I get a phone call just as I am about the put the boys to bed, or when I'm sitting down to have tea, I don't answer it. I will make a point of ringing or texting that person back but if it's going to interrupt something I want to do, or impact on time with my boys then I don't do it. Obviously, if I thought it was an emergency then I would answer it.

Choose how you spend your time carefully. Put yourself first sometimes. Your job is not to just be there for everyone else.

Remember...be brave and say "NO!"

"Daring to set boundaries is not about having the courage to love ourselves even when we risk disappointing others."

BRENE BROWN

Say "YES!"

I've found that one of the best ways to beat my anxiety and feel better about myself is to set small challenges outside of my comfort zone. For example, I used to be very self-conscious and would never leave the house without a full face of make-up and my hair done. I wanted so desperately to feel comfortable in my own skin and not worry what others thought of me, so I set myself the challenge of going to the local shop without any make-up. The first time I did it, I must admit, I scurried in and out, determined not to give anyone eye contact!

Once I got home and realised people hadn't left screaming because a hideous monster had just entered the shop, I felt slightly more relaxed! I tried something out of my comfort zone and nothing happened! There were no terrible consequences. I noticed people just seemed more concerned with what they were doing and weren't interested in me at all! Once I'd been to the shop, I then tried not putting any make-up on when friends came round; then I did the school run with no make-up on and wet hair. It has got to the point now where I am comfortable being me and don't feel the need to try and impress people.

If something scares me now, I automatically get a rush of excitement. I know that I definitely need to do that thing because, from experience, when I've pushed myself outside of my comfort zone, I have felt a massive sense of achievement and learnt a lot about myself. *Don't let fear hold you back - fear is normal. It means you are about to learn something.* Opportunities arise for a reason. Say 'yes' before you have chance to think about it and let your anxiety take hold. The feeling of regret lasts longer than the fear.

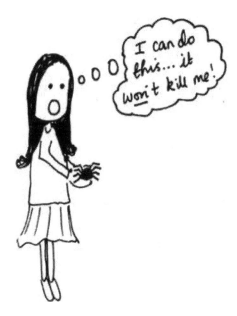

Remember...fear is temporary. Fear is not going to kill you. You can push through it. You'll feel incredible when you've come out of the other side!

Projection

Learning about projection when I was training to be a coun-sellor was something that really gave my self-esteem and con-fidence a boost. This will stay with me forever and has really stopped me from worrying about whether people like me or not (something which I've spent my life agonising over!). Have you ever met someone for the first time and within a few minutes of being in their company, you've had a strong feeling that you don't like them? You know that you don't even know them, but there is something about them which is really rub-bing you up the wrong way? Well, this could be projection at work. When we have a strong negative reaction to someone, it could be that they have something about them that we wish we had ourselves.

As I said, I was painfully shy up until a few years ago when I started on my personal growth journey. Even as an adult, if I was in a group situation, I could not speak in front of others. People that found that easy and always had something to say, irritated the life out of me! I would dislike them instantly, thinking they were arrogant, loud-mouthed, opinionated, attention-seeking floozies! Most of the time I hadn't even spoken to these people, so my judgement was a tad on the harsh side to say the least!

After learning about projection, I realised that they had something that I wish I had. Confidence! Opinions! I was jealous! I wish I could confidently share my thoughts and opinions to a group of people who I barely knew. It irritated the life out of me that they could do it so effortlessly and I couldn't. I was intimi-dated by them.

Nowadays, if I get the feeling that someone doesn't like me and I know that they don't know me well enough to truly form a judgement, then I don't worry about it like I used to. I now think, *"What are you seeing in me that you wish you had? What are you finding intimidating about me?"* It has helped me to distance myself from the negativity and respectfully give it back to them where it belongs. I know it's their issue and one that they need to reflect on. I know I can't physically do anything to change their opinion of me. If anything, instead of letting it upset me, I find myself being overly polite! I almost set myself a challenge – you WILL like me!!

Out of five people that you meet, one will like you straight away, one will have an automatic dislike to you and the other three aren't that bothered and haven't really made up their mind! Don't waste your time and energy worrying about the people who don't like you – they probably never will, but that's not your fault.

Remember...if someone doesn't like you, be flattered!

Fake it until you make it

I am more confident now than I've ever been. Faking being confident helped me to overcome my fear of speaking in front of people. The confident people I once hated became my teachers (without knowing it). I thought carefully about what they did that made them seem confident. I observed new confident people I met, looking for the answers I needed to help me transform. I studied how they walked, talked, held their head, facial expressions, what they did with their hands and I copied it (in Neuro-linguistic programming terms, this is called modelling).

I looked at my own body language and noticed how much I fiddle when I'm nervous. I pick at the skin around my fingers, I play with my hair, I wobble my foot. All these things seemed to exacerbate how I was feeling. As I mentioned earlier, your physiology (the way you move your body) impacts and exaggerates your emotions. I have learnt since studying NLP that all the things I do when I am nervous are my strategy. Everyone has a set pattern of behaviour, a strategy, for different emotions. As soon as I carry out that exact set of behaviours, my body is sending signals to my brain, telling it that it's time to be nervous. I realised that I needed to break that pattern. I noticed that confident people tended to walk with their heads held higher, they gave good eye contact, they talked more slowly, they generally smiled more and they were still and had a calmness about them (there were certainly no wobbly feet!). What confident people do you know? What do they do that's different to you?

So, not only are you going to do some modelling, try raising your sternum (chest bone) just ever so slightly as you're talking and walking. It will automatically give you a boost in confidence.

I love the idea that Beyonce has her alter-ego. For those of you that don't know, before Beyonce goes on stage and to help get her ready mentally to put on a good show, she gets herself into the role of a diva-like character she created called 'Sasha Fierce'. A great way of faking it until you make it! I wonder what your uber-confident alter-ego would be called?!

Remember...the more you act as if you were that confident person, before you know it, that is exactly who you will become!

In summary...

You are as important as anyone else that has walked the planet. Looking after yourself should not be a luxury and something you do on special occasions. Self-care should be at the forefront of your mind every day. If you want others to treat you with care and respect, then you have to give it to yourself first. Having firm boundaries and clear expectations about what you will and will not tolerate are the best ways to demonstrate to people how you want to be treated. We treat others how they allow us to, no matter who we are.

I consider myself to be a generally pleasant person, however, with my mum I can find myself being quite grumpy and at times rude. Unconsciously, I know she doesn't have firm boundaries and she will accept whatever I say to her. She allows people to treat her badly and unfortunately, they often do. We need to love ourselves enough that we demand respect from others. If you take anything away from this section, let it be a reflection on the following...

If you loved yourself, how would you treat yourself? If you loved yourself, how would you expect others to treat you?

CARE FOR YOUR BODY

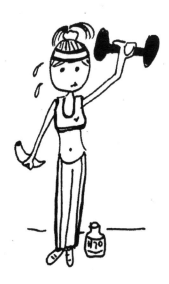

"Take care of your body, it's the only place you have to live."

Care For Your Body

By now, you'll have learned new ways of gaining control over your mood and emotions. However, as we've said, this can sometimes be difficult to maintain. As soon as you get run down, poorly or tired, this control feels like it goes out of the window. You are in a process of learning a whole new way of thinking and being and, at times, this is going to feel tiring and difficult. This next section is to show you how to raise your energy levels to help you to maintain your positive mood and attitude. You may be tempted to skip this section because it talks about the dreaded 'E' word (exercise!) and nutrition, but life is all about getting the balance right. You can't possibly maintain your new positive, energised way of life if you live off take-aways and spend your time on the sofa, watching mind-numbing reality TV. If you want to make lasting changes in your life, you really do need to shake things up and be open to trying new things. I know what some of you are thinking, "I just don't do exercise. I'm not one of those types of people. It's not me". Well, remember this is all about creating a new you.

You can be whoever you want to be!

Commit to caring for yourself

We've talked about the impact that incorporating positive affirmations into your daily practice can make. To really enhance this practice and help improve your feelings of self-worth, you need to change your actions as well as your thoughts. Care for yourself how you would if you believed that you were good enough; if you deserved to be happy; if you were a good person; if you loved yourself.

Commit to treating yourself to a monthly massage or having your nails done; taking time to meet a friend for coffee or buying a new top. Caring for yourself doesn't have to cost a lot of money– it can be anything that makes you feel good, like: treating yourself to a relaxing, candle-lit bath; going for a long, country walk; spending longer exfoliating in the shower; treating yourself to your favourite chocolate bar; booking that appointment at the dentist!

It's these things that can easily fall off the to-do list as we convince ourselves that we just haven't got the time or money for it this month. If you start putting these things off, before you know it two years will have passed, and you'll need even more work done at the dentist and you'll need even more money and time! Why put yourself through unnecessary torture?! Keeping on top of the dentist, eye tests, smear tests and other regular medical/health appointments should be your priority. If you don't look after yourself, who will?

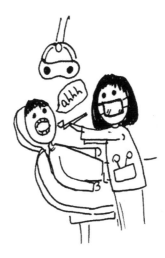

Make a promise to yourself to get on the phone and book the appointments you've been putting off for so long.

Remember...self-care is a necessity.

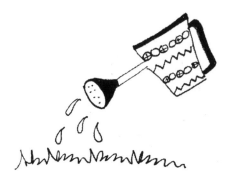

"The grass is always greener where you water it."

Run, run, run!

I absolutely hated exercise up until a few years ago. I never liked it at school – I always had a sick note, always having time-of-the-month-lady-issues! I now couldn't do without it. It's the one thing that has the most positive impact on my mood and ability to cope with my ever-changing emotions.

I remember so clearly the day that I decided that I needed to run. It was six years ago when I was coming out of the other side of my depression. My husband had persuaded me to go to the gym with him as he had a guest pass. I went and it was all fine but on the way home I suddenly said, "STOP THE CAR!! I NEED TO GET OUT AND RUN!!" My husband thought I was going mad! I ran home (it was only ½ a mile), with my husband driving up and down the road past me to make sure that I wasn't having a mental breakdown! I burst through the door, feeling as though I'd completed a marathon. I was bright red, panting and felt as though I was going to be sick, but I did it! Running then became something that I needed. I needed the space. I needed to feel the wind on my face. After that day, I found myself having an urge to stick my head out of my bathroom window, close my eyes and breathe in the fresh air. Odd I know! I felt for the first time in a long time that I could properly breathe – that I was alive. Running became a big part of my life and an important part of my recovery.

You might be thinking, "Well, I'm no runner! I'd never be able to do that". If I can do it, anyone can! I used to drive past runners and think, first of all, "What is wrong with *those people*?!" and secondly, "I wish I could be one of *those people*". Now I am! You can be too! Start off small by power walking and when you're ready, break out into a little jog, even if it's for 30 seconds. I tried alternating walking and running in between lampposts. Keep repeating this and, before you know it, you'll be able to run ½ mile, then 1 mile, then 5k and then 10k! Your stamina builds up so quickly. For me, running is the best medicine for low energy;

anxiety; shaking off a bad mood; helping me to visualise my goals; gaining clarity for relationship issues. There are so many benefits for your mental health as well as helping you to feel fitter and possibly lose weight as a bonus.

Remember...you can be whoever you want to be! Everyone has to start somewhere.

Daily exercise

If you think running really isn't your thing or maybe you have an injury or disability that would stop you from running, that's OK. You have to find your *thing*. For some people it's going to the gym, for others it's yoga or cycling. Whatever you prefer, I recommend that you start your day with 30 minutes of exercise, whatever that may be.

You may be saying, "I haven't got time to do that!" I would answer, "Oh, yes you have! Get up earlier!" If we value something enough, we will make time for it. We all have the same number of hours in the day. There's no better feeling than running through the streets at 5am before other people have woken up. The sense of achievement I get from that is unreal. I think, "I could be in bed right now, but instead I'm choosing to run 4 miles before breakfast!" Starting your day feeling proud of yourself is going to help set up your day just nicely.

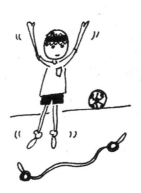

Even just setting yourself the challenge of walking 10,000 steps a day can have a big impact on your physical and mental health. Depending on what job you do, I know 10,000 steps can feel like a lot. If I didn't run in the morning, then I wouldn't clock up many steps because I literally sit down all day seeing clients. The most I move is to walk to the filing cabinet and then to the door to let clients in. Due to this, I try and fit exercise in where I can. Dr. Rangan Chatterjee calls this 'movement snacking', which I love. For me this can look like the following:

- Running on the spot with high knees while I'm waiting for the kettle to boil

- Sumo squats while I'm drying my hair

- Tricep dips on my settee while I am waiting for my next client to arrive

- Bouncing on the trampoline while testing the boys on their spellings

- Running up the stairs instead of walking

- Taking extra trips up the stairs if I'm moving things to another floor

I wonder...where you could squeeze in your movement snacks? Make a promise to yourself to be more active.

Five second rule

Now you've probably heard about the 5 second rule relating to dropping your food on the floor and it being OK to eat as long as you've picked it up within 5 seconds? Well, this is slightly different! There's a great book by Mel Robbins called the '5 Second Rule' relating to achieving your goals. I use this principle most mornings as soon as I wake up. As you know, I run most mornings, but I'll let you into a little secret…most mornings I don't actually want to go! I go because I know how good it is for my body and, more importantly my mind, but it's not always something I am desperate to do. The idea is, if you think about doing a certain thing and give your brain more than 5 seconds before starting it, that's enough time for your brain to talk you out of it. It will come up with as many reasons as possible why you shouldn't do that thing and why it's not a priority for you right now. It wants you to be safe and going out and doing anything is risky! If I don't spring out of bed when my alarm goes off, then I'll start thinking…

"I am too tired – it'll be better for me to have another half an hour."

"I'll just go later." (which never happens!)

"I went yesterday, so it'll be OK to have a day off." etc. etc. etc!

I have an actual argument in my head which is painful! If I give in to the thoughts and don't go, then I feel off all day. I feel more tired. I am kicking myself all day thinking, "I SHOULD HAVE GONE FOR A RUN!" To combat this mental argument, I do what I can to stop the thoughts popping in at all. Quite often, I sleep in my running clothes so that when my alarm goes off, I can literally go straight away. I'll be able to put my trainers and high vis on straight away because I'll have laid them all out the night before. It only takes a minor delay, like not being able to find my headphones, to allow enough time for the excuses to creep in. So, when my alarm goes off in the morning, I give myself a mental countdown and say, "5,4,3,2,1 and GO!" As soon as I say "Go", I force myself to get up and I'm out the door and walking before I'm properly awake - before my brain has had a chance to realise what I am doing. I walk to the end of the street to allow myself to wake up a bit and then get running. By the time I'm home, I feel energised, alive and proud of myself. A great way to start the day! It's this feeling that motivates me to keep doing it.

Remember...motivation doesn't just come to you, you have to MAKE yourself do it and then the positive feeling you get helps to keep you motivated.

Find your motivation

In my opinion, the hardest part of anything is starting it (especially if you haven't got the right gear). For me, there is nothing more motivating than investing in new exercise things – whether that be running shoes, a new energy drink or technology, like a fitness tracker. My Fitbit has been a big motivator over the last few years. It has everything on it to help you create a healthier life. You can track your steps, calories, how much water you've drunk, how well you've slept, weight loss and, ladies, it can even help you track your monthly cycle. It can help you to connect with others by allowing you to invite your friends to compete in challenges.

It helps me to stay on track and helps to simplify things for me. I've tried many diets and detoxes over the years but what I've learnt is, that if your aim is to lose weight, you just need to make sure you are burning off more calories than you are eating. At times, I have been regimental with my food and have not wanted to eat certain foods if they're seen as 'bad'. I have deprived myself unnecessarily. If you are logging your exercise and calories burned on the Fitbit, then you'll most probably be able to see that you can eat that chocolate bar guilt-free, as actually you're still below your calories. Equally, if you want to eat the chocolate bar but you've not done much exercise that day, you'll be able to see how much it will put you over your calories and then you can make an informed choice about whether you want it or not.

You don't always have to be spending money to fuel your motivation though. There are free apps that can track your fitness; you can find a friend who would like to exercise with you and be your motivational buddy when you're tempted to slack off or you can make your own reward chart, if that sort of thing works for you. When I went to Slimming World, I was given a picture of a hot air balloon. Every time I lost a pound, I could colour in a section. When the whole balloon was coloured in, it meant I'd have lost a stone in total. I love things like that! What could support you to stay on track?

Whatever you do to find your motivation just try and stay off the scales! In my experience, they have the opposite effect. If you've been 'good' all week and still not lost any weight, it is completely devastating! It makes me want to stuff my face with more chocolate! Scales are not always the most accurate way of measuring your progress if your goal is to lose weight. We can put weight on at the time of the month, if we're carrying excess water. Weight doesn't always mean fat. My weight hasn't really changed in the last two years, but my body is a completely different shape and size. I probably weigh more as I have muscle now (not much, but definitely some!) Taking photos of yourself or measuring your body with a tape measure can be a more accurate way of seeing if you're on the right track. Get rid of those scales today!

Remember...stop torturing yourself – motivate yourself in a healthy way!

Lymphasising

Tony Robbins has a great way of increasing his energy levels and keeping him in a peak state while he is on stage. He bounces on a trampoline! I used to think it was having more sleep or eating certain foods that gave me more energy. Although this can certainly help, it's actually the quality of the cells in your body that determine your energy levels. Bouncing, rebounding or lymphasising, whatever you'd like to call it, is brilliant for giving you an energy boost. As you jump, the pull of gravity makes your cells collide together which challenges their structure, making them stronger. The stronger your cells, the better able you are to fight off diseases and the healthier you are. There are many other benefits to bouncing, such as:

- improved posture
- better muscle tone
- improved co-ordination
- better balance
- stronger heart muscle
- stimulating the lymphatic drainage system which rids your body of toxins, bacteria and cancer cells
- improved mood (especially if you bounce to some of your favourite music!)

As soon as I came back from seeing Tony Robbins, I went out the next day and bought myself a mini trampoline and I haven't looked back since. I have one downstairs in our kitchen so that while I'm waiting for the dinner to cook or listening to the boys read, I can bounce.

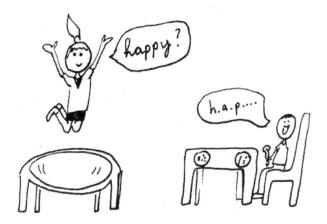

I also have one in the kitchen in my office that I use in between clients to give me an energy boost, to help make sure I'm on top form. The key is not to worry about what other people think. I often get asked why I have a trampoline, followed by a look that suggests I may have sprouted an extra head! Do whatever you need to do to feel better.

I wonder...what it would feel like if you put on your energising playlist and let yourself have fun; hands in the air and bounce like you were 5 again!

Yoga

Yoga has been my saviour at times. It's like meditation and exercise all in one. Win-win! It has helped to calm my anxious mind; take time out from the hustle and bustle of life; start the day doing something for myself that I'm proud of; unwind after a stressful day; tone my body; build strength - the benefits are endless. Don't worry, you don't need to be as flexible as a gymnast to do it. There are lots of free programmes that you can follow on YouTube that will suit your level. My favourite is 'Yoga with Adriene' – she's obviously very skilled at what she does but doesn't take herself too seriously, which I really like as it helps me to relax more. You'll wobble and definitely shake to start with, but it's amazing how quickly you build your strength and flexibility. Give it a go! Namaste!

**Remember...it is about trying something
new and finding your thing.**

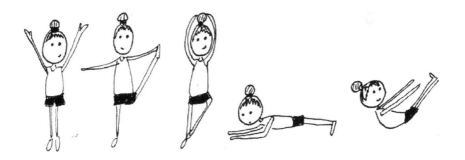

Connect with Mother Nature

One of my absolute favourite things to do is to go for a walk in the woods or countryside when the sun is shining. I love to be outdoors. I love to feel the breeze on my face and the warm sun on my skin. I am really not designed to be a sun lover though with my ginger hair and pale skin. I love it but it definitely doesn't like me very much! Every year I notice a negative change in my mood as the Autumn months make an appearance. It is quite common for people to suffer with SAD – Seasonal Affective Disorder - especially, if you work long hours in an office or a factory where you are going to work and coming home in the dark.

Spending time in the sun can really boost your mood and make you feel better. Sunlight also prompts the production of Vitamin D which has a number of health benefits, such as, healthier bones, potential weight loss, a decreased risk of certain cancers and improved sleep. It is worth mentioning that I have had a number of clients explain that they have been struggling with low mood and a lack of energy, and they've been unable to figure out why they feel that way. Upon visiting the doctor, blood tests have revealed a vitamin D deficiency and as soon as they've started taking vitamin D supplements, they have noticed a significant improvement in their symptoms. I found it astonishing that something as simple as a vitamin deficiency could have such an impact on mental health. I now regularly suggest that my clients get an MOT check at the doctors to make sure that their emotions and moods are not related to something physical.

There are many benefits to being outside full stop. I love to get out after it's been raining and watch my boys and my crazy dog jumping in and out of the muddy puddles and then going home, all rosy-cheeked for a sneaky hot chocolate and marshmallows! According to the University of East Anglia spending time in nature reduces the risk of type II diabetes, cardiovascular disease, premature death, stress and high blood pressure. They found that populations with higher levels of exposure to the outdoors are more likely to report good overall health.

It is thought that the most beneficial time of the day to absorb sunlight is first thing in the morning. Starting your day with a 20-minute walk in nature, soaking up natural day light helps your body to release serotonin, a chemical that makes you happier. It also really helps to reset your circadian rhythm to get a good nights' sleep.

Please make sure that if you're out and about in the sun, you have sun cream on, are covered up as much as possible, limit your time in direct sunlight and avoid midday sun, if at all possible.

Remember...get outdoors as much as possible to heal your body and mind.

Early bird

We've all used the excuse at some point in our lives that we just simply don't have enough time. I was very guilty for filling my days with meaningless rubbish and said many times that I didn't have time for things like exercise, relaxing, seeing friends or preparing healthy meals etc. Time, or lack of it, was my excuse for everything! The truth is that you'll make time for the things that you value in life. I always made the time to watch Big Brother or some other rubbish reality programme, but I didn't have time to read a book. I always found 10-15 minutes to scroll mindlessly through social media, but I didn't have 10 minutes to spare a day for meditation and relaxation. It's crazy when I look back now! If you love and care for yourself, then you'll want to fill your days with things that you know are going to be of benefit to you. I now rarely watch TV in an evening. I exercise, read a book or spend quality time chatting to my husband.

Getting up an hour earlier each day can have a massive impact on the quality of your life. If you got up an hour earlier for a year, then you would gain an extra...

30 hours per month (equivalent to nearly 1 ½ days)

365 hours per year (equivalent to more than 15 days)

1,825 hours over 5 years (equivalent to 75 days!!!!!)

I wonder...what you could do with that extra time?

You might be thinking, "Yes but, I need to have 8 hours of sleep every night". You indeed might. But many adults don't need that much – it's completely individual. It's more about getting good quality sleep rather than the quantity. In my experience, when I started getting up earlier, I felt more energised and didn't have the need for an afternoon nap, which is something I've done since being a teenager. I would highly recommend reading 'The 5am Club' by Robin Sharma. I now get up 5am every morning and do some form of exercise. I must admit that I felt like I had been hit by a bus for the first week of doing this, but it's surprising how quickly your body adapts. I now wake up every morning before my alarm goes off and I generally feel awake and ready to go. I have 3 ½ hours in the morning before I have to take the boys to school. We no longer rush around; everything is organised and I feel proud of myself before the day has really started.

You need to do what is right for you and your body, but using time as your excuse is no longer cutting it!

Remember...if you want to do something, you'll make the time!

Hour of power

We've talked about the importance of starting your day as positively as you can and the benefits of getting up earlier. If you can get up an hour earlier than usual, you can use this time to set you up for the rest of the day. Below is an example of how you could use, what Tony Robbins' calls your 'Hour of Power', to the full!

30 minutes of exercise – Whatever exercise you do, it's best to choose something that raises your heart rate and gets your blood pumping to give your body a real kickstart and get everything moving.

10 minutes of meditating – I either put on a relaxing piece of music that I like or I do Tony Robbins' Priming exercise (this can be found on YouTube or at www.tonyrobbins.com). Sometimes, I need silence so I just concentrate on my breathing and slowing everything down.

5 minutes of gratitude – I spend 5 minutes filling out my gratitude journal and creating a positive mindset for the day. I use 'The Daily Greatness Journal' by Lyndelle Palmer-Clarke, but it's just as effective to jot your thoughts down in a notebook.

5 minutes of visualisation – I spend 5 minutes reading my goals for the coming year and really soaking them up. I close my eyes and visualise what it would feel like to achieve them. I had a goal for finishing this book, which was to visualise standing in a shop, seeing people pick up my book and allow myself to feel the excitement and pride that I would feel if that happened. Visualising this was especially important to do when my self-doubt crept in and I wanted to give up on it.

5 minutes of affirmations – I type out my affirmations and put them in my journal so that I can read through them and repeat them to myself, again to help create a positive mind-set. My affirmations change every few weeks depending on what I need to hear and feel at that moment. For example, if I am lacking in confidence in my job then my affirmations might be...

I am professional

I am a kick-ass counsellor and coach

I am knowledgeable and skilled etc. etc.

My affirmations always end with, '*I am Claire f**king Reeves!*' to give me that extra bit of power and oomph! Try it for yourself. It's better than an energy drink and it has 0% sugar!

5 minutes of smoothie making – I make a healthy smoothie every day to take to my office with me so that if I'm hungry I won't be tempted to grab something. Also, it feels great to know that I'm spending my time doing something that's going to be good for my body. Being organised helps me to feel in control and powerful! I feel like I'm winning at life!

There is also a great book called 'The Miracle Morning' by Hal Elrod, which is very similar to the Hour of Power. He calls the elements of the Miracle Morning Life SAVERS which I love, where each letter of SAVERS represents a positive activity.

S = silence (meditating, breathing exercises)

A = affirmations

V = visualisation

E = exercise

R = reading (a few pages of something positive)

S = scribing (writing in a journal)

You can spend your hour in any way that suits you as long as you're immersed in positivity and are doing things that are good for your body and mind! My advice to you is try different things within your hour, try them in a different order and once you've found what works, repeat it until it is firmly part of your routine. It doesn't just have to be an hour either. I probably spend more like 90 minutes, especially if I do a longer run. You are completely in control, there is no right or wrong.

Remember...the first hour of the morning is the rudder of the day.

The importance of sleep

Getting a good night's sleep is so important. When you've rested and had enough sleep then everything feels easier! When you've had too little sleep (or too much in some cases) things that wouldn't normally bother you, feel enormous. It feels harder to stay in control where your emotions are concerned. There are other benefits to getting the right amount of good, quality sleep, such as:

- improved concentration and memory
- the ability to be more creative
- increased energy levels
- maintaining a healthy weight by making better food choices
- decreased risk of illnesses, such as heart disease, stroke, diabetes, arthritis
- decreased stress levels
- being less accident prone
- improved immune system
- decreased risk of Alzheimer's
- live longer!

When we sleep, a major clean-up process begins to happen in our bodies called autophagy. Imagine it's like clearing up the mess after you've had a big party. Autophagy works by mopping up any waste that has accumulated in our cells during the day. It helps to clear out and repair damaged cells. Our body literally eats itself -it strips the dead cells of parts it needs to make new cells. It's our very own internal recycling system.

A study carried out by the University of Rochester Medical Center (URMC) found that the brain's cells shrivel up by 60% while we sleep to allow gaps to open up between our nerve cells so that any waste can be dealt with. This is one of the reasons why we still burn off a lot of energy while we sleep, because our body goes into crazy cleaning mode. This waste removal is important as it helps to protect our body against cancer, infections, aging, memory loss and inflammatory diseases. So, sleeping actually does help us to live longer.

I don't think there is anything more frustrating than not being able to sleep. If you suffer with anxiety, then having trouble sleeping is almost inevitable. You may struggle to switch your brain off and have trouble falling to sleep. The day's events will whirl around your head and you start to predict what may happen the following day. There are many things you can do to help improve your ability to fall asleep and stay asleep.

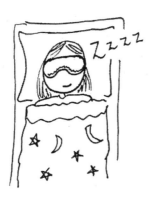

Tips for improving sleep:
- Stick to a sleep schedule (even on weekends)
- Practise a relaxing bedtime ritual
- Exercise daily (preferably in the morning)
- Get out in the fresh air and get plenty of natural sunlight during the day
- Avoid napping in the middle of the day
- Make sure that your bedroom is dark
- Make sure that the temperature in your room is suitable – cooler is better
- Sleep on a comfortable mattress and pillows

- Reduce alcohol consumption – although it knocks you out, it lessens sleep quality
- Avoid caffeine after lunchtime
- Try not to eat at least three hours before bedtime
- Turn off electronic screens at least an hour before you go to bed
- Don't take your phone into your bedroom at night-time – use something else as your alarm
- Drink camomile tea before bed
- Meditate or practise relaxation strategies before bed
- Put on relaxing music and leave it on throughout the night (so that if you wake up in the night it will help you to drift off again)
- Try ASMR (Autonomic Sensory Meridian Response) – listening to everyday sounds such as rain, waves, paper rustling, hair being brushed – again there are many videos on YouTube
- Remove clocks from your sleep space where possible (if you wake up in the night and look at the clock, this can cause anxiety. You may worry that you've got to get up soon and get stressed about being tired the next day)
- If you wake up in the night to go to the toilet, avoid putting on the light – walk like a zombie and try to remain half asleep
- Write in a journal before bed to empty your mind of anything that is troubling you

Did you know the amount of sleep you need varies depending on your age? It's a scientific fact that babies and teenagers need a lot more sleep than adults. However, if you are getting considerably less than eight hours of sleep most nights, you may become sleep deprived. Sleep deprivation is dangerous. Driving after having less than five hours sleep is as dangerous as drink-driving. Your concentration is reduced, your reactions are slower, and your decision making is impaired.

It's also worth noting that the time of day in which we need to sleep changes in relation to our life stage. We all know of a teenager who is up until the early hours of the morning and then sleeps in until lunchtime. It isn't that they're lazy. Teenagers' circadian rhythms are slightly different to that of adults and they generally feel the need to sleep later than their parents. Needing to sleep later isn't the same as sleeping more though. Research has shown that people who regularly sleep more than nine hours per night are more likely to die early! The same goes for people who regularly had less than six hours sleep a night. Sleeping between 6-8 hours per night is perfect. Listen to your body. It knows what it needs.

Remember...make sleep your priority.

"Sleep is the glue that holds your glitter together."

Back to basics

We all know what we 'should' or 'shouldn't' be eating, but often the little voice in our head is shouting too loud for us to ignore and before we know if we've eaten a giant bar of Cadbury's Fruit and Nut, had 8 cups of coffee and finished the day with a chippy tea. As great as these things are, the saying, 'everything in moderation,' is extremely important. For you to maintain your energy levels and keep the positive wheels of your brain turning, you need to be putting the right fuel into your body. Anything you put in your body, other than pure water, needs energy and water to break it down and turn it into something useful.

Here's a reminder of the things we all know but sometimes forget...

Get More Of...

1. Water
• You should ideally drink ½ your body weight in water each day. For example, if you weigh 200lbs (just over 14 stones) then you should drink 100 ounces of water which is the equivalent to 6.25 pints or 2.96 litres. Keep it simple - if you're drinking more than 2 litres of water per day then you're doing great.
• Ideally do not go longer than 20 minutes without sipping water. You can get brilliant apps on your phone that you can set to give you a little reminder to take a sip.
• You're most toxic and dehydrated first thing in the morning – make it a habit to drink a glass of water before you get out of bed.
• Drink a glass of water before eating a meal as this helps with the digestive process.
• Try adding a fresh lemon to your water to help clear out toxins and help with weight loss.

2. Clean, healthy food

· Try to eat more fresh fruit and vegetables that are full of water (i.e. lettuce, melon, broccoli, carrots) as your body will find it easier to break these foods down. A great way to make sure you're eating plenty of fruit and vegetables is to try and eat foods of all the colours of the rainbow. If your plate is mainly made up of beige foods then that's probably not a great sign that you are getting a healthy balance!

· The more green vegetables you can eat the better. These will help to balance your body's pH levels and make it more alkaline which is better for helping your cells to thrive. If your body is too acidic then it will start to fight itself which is obviously not good! If your body doesn't have the alkaline level that it needs, it will put more in the body by using calcium from your bones – again, definitely not good! You can test the alkalinity of your body by buying pH testing strips (you can get these from Amazon for a few pennies). Ideally your pH levels should be around a 7 – balanced in the middle of acid and alkaline.

· More and more people seem to be gluten intolerant. Over the last few years, the free-from section in most supermarkets has gone from a shelf to a whole aisle! Humans evolved to eat whatever food was available - their diet being made up mainly of seasonal fruits and vegetables, meat, eggs, nuts and seeds. In terms of evolution, wheat has been a fairly new addition to our diets and we have not necessarily evolved enough to process it properly without it having an adverse effect on our gut. If you suffer from bloating, excess wind, IBS – try cutting out gluten for a month to see if it makes a difference.

· Nowadays, sugar addiction is a very real thing. Spikes in our blood sugar levels, light up the same part of our brain that is involved in pleasure and reward. It is the same part that lights up in people with drug addictions. If you feel the need to eat every two hours; struggle to concentrate mid-morning; feel shaky/dizzy in between meals; have an afternoon slump; rely on caffeine to give you an energy boost or crave sweet things in between meals then you could very well have a sugar addiction.

Too much sugar in the diet has been linked to weight gain, type II diabetes, acne, depression, cancer and accelerated aging. Not to mention being grumbled at by the dentist! Try cutting down on your sugar intake and notice your taste buds change. I used to drink tea with 2 sugars and then cut out sugar completely. If someone accidently put sugar in my tea now, I would probably spit it out because it would taste disgusting! I wonder if that has happened to you?

• Watch your portion sizes! A jacket potato should be no bigger than a computer mouse! I didn't know this! I love a jacket!

• Eat in a relaxed, calm state to help with digestion. No more eating meals standing up in the kitchen while you're trying to do a million other jobs!

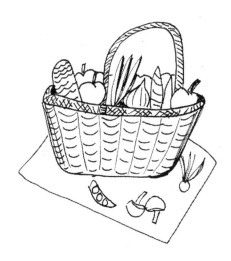

Cut Down On (Or Eliminate)...

1. Caffeine
• It triggers the release of adrenaline, which is responsible for the fight or flight response. It raises your heart rate and blood pressure; can cause rapid breathing; it makes you hyper-alert and therefore can worsen anxiety as it mimics the symptoms of it.

- Caffeine stimulates the kidneys to secrete water which makes you more dehydrated.
- It inhibits the enzymes that support memory function.
- It speeds up the activity of the colon and can cause digestive issues.
- The level of caffeine in your body only drops by half in 4-6 hours. If you're having caffeine in the afternoon/evening, it's very likely that this will be having an impact on your sleep. Caffeine blocks the release of adenosine which sends sleep signals to your brain, it therefore tricks your body into thinking its alert and awake. If you are not ready to give up coffee altogether, try and drink it early in the morning.

2. Meat
- Hearing this has put me off eating meat for life! As a teenager, I used to be a vegetarian for ethical reasons but if I'm honest at the time, I couldn't do without a Greggs sausage roll, McDonald's Big Mac and KFC! There are still times when I could murder a sausage roll! Were you aware the moment an animal is killed, it goes into a decaying stage? The flesh of the animal grows more and more bacteria, making it harder for the body to digest and break it down. Therefore, it can really sap you of your energy. You may have noticed that after eating a big roast Sunday dinner or a large steak you've then felt the need to sleep all afternoon – this is why.
- Studies show that eating a high meat-based diet can increase the risk of heart disease and cancers.

3. Dairy
- Animal proteins increase the acidity of the body which pulls calcium from the bones, weakening them, increasing the risk of osteoporosis.
- You may not realise this but you can get all the calcium you

need in your diet from other foods such as soya, rice milk, almond milk, broccoli, kale etc.
• Eating and drinking dairy products can lead to the body producing excessive amounts of mucus. Gross! This then sits in the intestines and forms a lining making it harder for them to absorb the nutrients needed. This can lead to fatigue as your body has to work harder to break down the food.

4. Alcohol/drugs/nicotine
• You don't need me to tell you about the dangers of putting these in your body. They are pure poison. If you loved and cared for your body, then you would want to treat it with respect. You only have one! Look after it!

All these things help to create an acidic environment in your body which is conducive for the growth of viruses, bacteria, yeast and fungus! Not nice!

I'm not trying to preach and tell you that you need to completely cut out the above. It is just about being aware of what you're putting into your body. Is it going to be good for you or do you harm? Is it going to cleanse your body or clog you up? It seems a bit contradictory to be filling your mind with positive affirmations; being kind to yourself; being aware of your strengths; doing things to show that you love yourself, but then feeding your body poison.

Remember...for this transformation to be successful and for you to get to where you want to be, then it needs to be a whole body and mind approach.

Healthy gut, healthy mind

I truly believe to achieve wellness, a whole-body approach is needed. This can be evidenced in what is known as, the gut-brain axis. The health of the gut and the brain are closely linked. You may have heard the gut being referred to as the 'second brain'? That is why. They are in constant communication, connected together by the vagus nerve.

Our gut is responsible for the production of the neurotransmitter and hormone serotonin. Low amounts of serotonin in the body are often linked to anxiety, depression and low mood. Serotonin is also responsible for regulating digestive secretions, the perception of pain and nausea, metabolism, appetite, concentration, body temperature and the sleep-wake cycle. It can also been found to be involved in conditions such as IBS (Irritable Bowel Syndrome). Research has shown the production of serotonin can be affected by the health of the bacteria found in our gut.

Inside our gut we have 100 trillion micro-organisms, which are a mixture of bacteria, viruses and fungi, collectively known as microbiome. More and more research has shown that the microbiome influences mental health. The microbiome is made up of 'good' and 'bad' bacteria. If the balance is off and you have more unhealthy bacteria, then you are more likely to develop inflammatory diseases, obesity and mental health issues.

So...what does all this mean in a nutshell?

If you are fuelling your body with unhealthy foods and drinks... the bacteria in your gut will become more unhealthy...which will inhibit the production of serotonin...which will impact your mental health. It is all connected.

There's good news though. You can improve the health of your microbiome by...

- Taking probiotics and eating fermented foods
- Eating prebiotic fibres which can be found in foods such as bananas, garlic, onions, asparagus
- Eating less sugars and sweeteners
- Reducing stress levels
- Avoid taking antibiotics unnecessarily
- Exercising regularly
- Getting plenty of sleep
- Eating a plant-based diet

If you wish to find out more about this, there is a great book called, 'Activate your vagus nerve', by Dr. Navaz Habi.

Remember...you are what you eat.

"The food you eat can either be the most powerful form of medicine or the slowest form of poison."

Mini-fasts

When our body is digesting food, it is in a natural state of stress, as it's working hard to break everything down to take what it needs to function. Many of us are guilty of grazing – a knob of cheese here, a handful of Maltesers there. The more we put in our bodies, the harder it has to work, the less energy it has reserved for other things, like our keeping our immune system healthy or helping us to manage our emotions.

Our bodies are not designed to be constantly eating and digesting. It is a habit that humans have got in to through fitting eating in around the working day. We've all been told that we should eat three meals a day. Actually, our digestive systems, the same as our nervous systems, are designed to be switched on for a period when needed but then have a period of rest. If you think back to caveman times again, we would feast on the hunt but then we might go for a few days with little to eat whilst waiting for the next big meal to be brought home. We have almost trained our bodies to be hungry at certain times. I know I could tell the time by my stomach!

So, what is the answer to this?

•   Know the difference between eating because you're hungry and eating because you're bored. I like that Dr Rangan Chatterjee describes this has having an 'itchy mouth!' I completely get that – sometimes I just fancy eating. I like eating!

•   Try to limit your eating to a twelve-hour window, maybe between 7am and 7pm, so that your body has a long period of rest ready to start again the next day.

•   Stick to drinking water or green tea outside of your twelve-hour window.

What are the benefits of mini-fasts?

· This mini-fasting approach (also known as intermittent fasting) is thought to encourage weight loss as fasting for 10-16 hours can cause the body to turn its fat into energy.

· The body generally functions better when it has the same rhythm so try and stick to the same 12 hours if possible.

· As mentioned in the earlier section, a process called autophagy happens when you're asleep to clean up any damaged cells and get rid of toxins. Fasting can help accelerate this process. In the absence of food, the body then turns to its stores and starts to eat itself which helps to lower blood pressure, reduce inflammation in the body, boost brain function and lower cholesterol.

I wonder...are you hungry or have you just got an itchy mouth??

Green tea

If you would like to cut down on caffeine but you enjoy a hot drink, then green tea makes a great alternative. Please be aware that green tea does still contain caffeine, so it's best to buy the de-caffeinated version. On that note, many people don't realise that de-caffeinated coffee still contains caffeine. De-caf doesn't mean no-caf so just be aware.

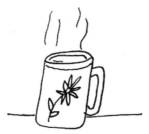

Green tea is full of antioxidants and nutrients that are good for your body. Regularly drinking green tea can have the following health benefits:

- Reduces risk of heart disease
- Lowers blood pressure
- Reduces cholesterol levels
- Reduces inflammation in cases of arthritis
- Improves bone density
- Inhibits the growth of some bacteria in the mouth, improving dental health and reducing bad breath
- Improves memory and brain function
- Lowers risk of cancer by reducing inflammation in the body
- Can help with weight loss

Remember...small healthy choices will add up to be big changes.

Cold showers – Brrrrrrrrr!

This is the best-worst thing I've tried! I must admit this was one of the suggestions from the Tony Robbins' 'Unleash the Power Within' weekend and it's taken me a year to try it! I love boiling hot showers and I just couldn't face it. I hate being cold! My husband thinks I'm some sort of lizard as I gravitate towards the sun and heat. However, cold showers are proven to have an amazing effect on your health and wellbeing. So, what are the benefits? Why would you want to put yourself through this torture?! There are many benefits:

- Increased energy levels
- Increased resilience levels
- Improved mood
- Improved skin and hair
- Weight loss
- Increased fertility
- Improved circulation
- Increased immunity
- Rids body of toxins
- Aids recovery after exercise
- Improves sleep

It really does work – but the torture takes some getting used to. Good luck with this one!

I wonder...how long could you stick it in the cold?!

In summary...

For change to be lasting and to create your magical days, you really do need to take a mind-body-spirit approach, as everything is connected. Making changes to your physical health can have such a huge impact on your emotional health. You might find though that as soon as you start to change your mindset and develop more self-love, you will naturally want to change how you treat your body. As I've said previously, if you truly cared for yourself, would you want to smoke and fill your lungs with harmful chemicals? If you cared about yourself, would you be happy living on a diet of takeaways?

Where your body is concerned, I have found that changing too many things all in one go can be hard to stick to. I would start with one thing and see if this makes a difference to how you feel emotionally, your energy levels, quality of sleep etc. I have been guilty for being a bit of a food Nazi at times and have denied myself of things that I really like. You've heard it a thousand times...it's everything in moderation. Life is for living too! If having a glass of wine on a Friday and Saturday night with your meal brings you pleasure, and it doesn't impact you negatively then continue to do so, if it feels right for you. Sometimes however, it is useful to start with cutting everything out that could be the culprit of making you feel lousy. When I decided to follow a vegan diet, after seeing Tony Robbins, I felt amazing but because I had made such a drastic change but I wasn't sure whether it was one particular thing that had made me feel better. After about 9 months, I started introducing different foods back into my diet (mainly because I could no longer live without cheese!) and it was then that I could identify anything that I was intolerant to or anything that made me have an energy slump after I'd eaten it. I now know that having the odd bit of cheese or dairy doesn't hurt me but 90% of the time I would choose an alternative. One thing I have not budged on is eating meat. After hearing about rotting flesh, I can't see me putting any sort of meat in my mouth again! Not even a Greggs sausage roll can tempt me!

Remember that everybody on the planet is different and every-

one's body is different and needs different things to help it to thrive. Find what works for you and you can't go far wrong.

I would suggest that if you intend to change your diet or anything that could impact your health that you seek advice from a GP first.

CREATE YOUR FUTURE

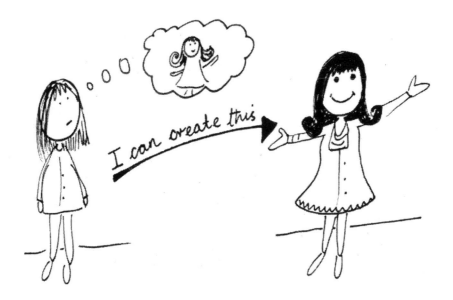

"Your future is created by what you do today, not tomorrow."

Create Your Future

Do you ever compare yourself to other people? How does that feel? Do you feel jealous, envious, insecure, annoyed, frustrated? Comparing yourself to others is never going to lead to positive emotions. Someone will always have something you don't have. Someone will always be better.

Scrolling through social media is the worst! How many times have you been mindlessly scrolling and then come across a post which has really p*ssed you off?! You notice that your friend has gone on another expensive holiday, or they look amazingly happy with their seemingly perfect family, or they're doing amazing 'mummin'. Remember, that all photos are just snapshots of a brief moment in time. Anyone can hold a smile for the time it takes to take the photo. The amount of times I've felt that I'm not a good enough mum, or my life is a bit rubbish because I've seen something in my newsfeed. The funny thing is though, when speaking to these 'perfect' people, they often tell a completely different story to what was portrayed in the picture. That's why I try not to go on social media – it's not real! I can make myself feel bad enough by criticising myself without having other people's 'perfect' lives being rubbed in my face!

Did you know that a study published in the Journal of Social and Clinical Psychology found that if you use social media less, you are less likely to suffer with depression and loneliness?

The thing is every single person on the planet is struggling in some way. Every single person is completely different. They have had different childhoods; different beliefs and values; different traumas; different metabolisms even! Comparing yourself to others is a futile task - no two people are the same. It would be like comparing a zebra with a horse. They might look very similar but live in very different environments and deal with very different threats. It's pointless. There's only one you, and YOU are the only one responsible for you and creating the life you want.

This might sound incredibly harsh, but are you unhappy with your size? Exercise and eat well! Hate your job? Change it! Want more money? Change your job/study/get a second job/ stop unnecessarily spending! I know it's not always that simple, but for most people it really is! Like I said earlier, it's time to stop blaming others, blaming your start in life and start taking responsibility. You only have one life. It's your responsibility to make sure that you're not wasting it. Every day is a gift. Make every day count!

So, you've mastered your thoughts, behaviour, have bags of energy – what next? It's time to start creating your future!

Goal setting

What is it that you want to achieve in life? Maybe you'd like to be thinner? Fitter? Have more money? Start your own business? Move house? Whatever your goals, you can achieve them. This isn't going to happen overnight, but every day you can take steps towards creating a better life. I would concentrate on no more than three goals at a time. You may just want to focus on one, depending on the size of the goal. It's OK to think about what you want to achieve, but I'd recommend that you write your goals down – it just feels a bit more formal and like you're making a commitment to yourself. I know you may be tempted to skip this part. I have read lots of self-help books and skipped the parts when it's asked me to do something! I've just expected my life to change through osmosis. However, if you seriously want to change your life, then you must put the work in. No short cuts!

I use the GROW model when I'm setting my goals. I have explained the model below using weight loss as an example, but you can apply this to any goal.

G = Goal – what is my goal?

Be as *specific* as possible. You can't just write that you want to lose weight because if you lose one pound then technically you've met your goal. Be specific. Write down *why* you want to achieve this goal. What are the *positive outcomes* of being your ideal weight? For example, your clothes will fit better; you'll feel more comfortable in your bikini; have more energy to run around with the children; you'll feel more confident etc.

R = Reality – what is my reality?

What do you currently weigh? Remember with weight, the scales aren't always the most accurate way of measuring your progress because if you increase your muscle mass then you might actually put weight on. I would take a photo of yourself and take measurements of your problem areas so that you can see that your body is changing. Also, write down the *negative consequences* of being this current weight/dress size, i.e. you get out of breath playing with your children; you find it hard to walk up the stairs; you couldn't fit in the harness on a ride at Alton Towers; you can't fit into your favourite jeans, etc. Also, could there be consequences in the future if you don't make this change? i.e. health issues, confidence issues affecting performance at work etc.

O = Options – what are your options?

This is where you write a list of all the things you could do to work towards achieving your goals. Make sure they're feasible. Start off small. For example, you might walk to work three out of the five days; you might go for a walk on your lunch break; you might join the gym; you might plan your meals for the week; you might sort out your fridge and cupboards to get rid of foods that you no longer want to eat regularly.

W = When – when are you going to achieve this goal by?

If your goal was to lose half a stone, what is a realistic time frame to achieve this by? At this point, think about potential stumbling blocks. What could get in the way of you achieving your goal? Maybe you have a weekend away planned. That's absolutely OK! Don't panic! You should still go and enjoy yourself, but it might be worth planning how you can still feel in control and make healthier choices. For example, pack some healthy snacks in your bag, so that you're not tempted to grab something that you would later regret.

Another thing to think about when writing your goal is to word it in a way that really connects with you on an emotional level. The best way of doing this is to write it as if you've already achieved it. Think about what this goal will look like when you've achieved it. Rather than writing, 'I am going to lose a stone', my goal would be...

'It is July 2020, I am lying on a beach in a white bikini showing off my toned stomach and thighs and feeling super confident in my own skin. My fitness levels have surpassed my expectations and I am feeling proud of what I have achieved'.

Doesn't this feel more compelling and exciting?!

Finally, it's good to tell your family and friends what your goal is. This helps to hold you to account but it may also help you to feel supported while you're making progress towards your goal, especially if its weight related. A considerate family member or friend probably wouldn't buy you a big box of chocolates for your birthday knowing you're focussing on losing weight. However, as a word of warning, sometimes people will deliberately try and sabotage your progress as they don't want you to change. Either because it makes them feel insecure that they will no longer be enough for you or because your change highlights where they are. Try your best to steer clear of negative people that could derail you.

Remember...this is your life. Stay focussed on what YOU want.

Review your progress

It's really important to regularly review your goal. What have you done so far to work towards it? What haven't you done? What is working? What is not working? I recommend that once a week you sit down and reflect on where you are with it. It might be that every Sunday morning as you have your breakfast and cup of green tea, you look back over the week and review how you've done. Then think about the coming week and what you can do to make progress; what obstacles you might face and how you will overcome them.

As I mentioned earlier, I use 'The Daily Greatness Journal' to help with my goal setting as there are sections in it for you to write your goals; create a plan of action and review them on a weekly basis. You don't need this though, but I recommend getting a notebook dedicated to tracking your progress. If you're taking photos of yourself, then maybe you could stick them in your book and create a timeline of your progress.

*Remember...reflecting on where you've been,
helps you to see where you need to go.*

"You can't go back to the beginning, but you can start where you are and change the ending."

C.S. LEWIS

Visualisation

We've talked about the Law of Attraction and how our thoughts are like magnets. Visualisation can really speed up the process of attracting positive things into your life. When you have written down your goals and you have it clear in your head where you want to get to, try incorporating some visualisation into your morning SAVERS or morning meditation. Close your eyes and imagine that you have achieved your goal. How does it feel? What do you look like? Where are you? Make sure that you are looking through your own eyes, as if you're really there. Look around you and take it all in. Visualising your goals isn't going to make them magically appear, but what it will do is start creating new neural networks in your brain which will allow you to be more open to the idea that this thing could actually happen. Once you are more open to it, your behaviour will become more in line with making it happen, as you start to say 'yes' to opportunities that you were once unaware of.

To start creating your dream life, try creating a Visualisation Board that you can look at every day. Fill the board with pictures of the body that you would like; your dream car; dream holiday destination, a blank cheque with an amount of money that you would like to attract. Again, as you look at them, feel how you would feel if you already had these things or if you knew for certain they were on their way. Whether these suggestions work or not to move you closer to your goals, it is a much more helpful thing to do than constantly focussing on what your life is lacking. When I made my board, I had pictures of a lady with toned arms; a red Renault Clio; a new tv; a holiday to Disneyland and a private practice with 5 clients. I focussed on the images every day; imagined me driving the car; stepping on to the plane to go to Disney with my toned arms; imagined opening my emails and seeing enquires from new clients. Within the year, I had achieved everything on the list, although my arms weren't quite as toned as the lady's in the picture, but I had definite muscle that wasn't there before.

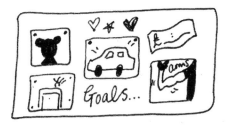

Remember...when you truly believe you can achieve, the magic starts to happen.

Leverage to change

To make a lasting change, you need to associate enough pain or pleasure to your goal that you no longer need to rely on willpower alone. I have a great example of this. A few years ago, some friends came around for dinner on New Year's Eve Eve and they brought dessert, which was a lovely chocolatey cheesecake. Now, up until this point I had been having issues with my belly so I was avoiding gluten and I thought I may have an intolerance to dairy. Everything in my bones was telling me that having the cheesecake would be a bad idea, but not wanting to offend our new friends, I had a slice. The next day I had a medical appointment in Nottingham which I'd been waiting for for months. I felt absolutely terrible before we set off – I had a blinding headache and I felt really sick, but off we went because I didn't want to miss the appointment.

Well, it went very wrong! I was sick nearly all the way there in a plastic bag which I didn't realise had a hole in it! I ended up holding the bag of sick out of the window as we were driving along, with it dripping down the side of the car. I turned up to the appointment covered in sick and looking like death. It was very embarrassing! As much as I still love cheesecake, there's absolutely no way I would have any now. I may have had a sickness bug and the cheesecake may not have been the culprit at all, but I'm not willing to take that chance. I have associated enough pain with cheesecake that willpower no longer plays a part!

This is what you need to do – associate enough pain with the idea of not changing that it is no longer an option - **YOU HAVE TO CHANGE.**

I'd like to share an exercise with you, but before we start, I must warn you that you may find this difficult as it's designed to open up difficult feelings. I wouldn't recommend it at the moment if you're already struggling emotionally and are feeling particularly vulnerable. I would come back to this one when you're feeling a bit stronger and more in control.

For this exercise, you'll need a pen and paper. You will need a quiet place where you won't be interrupted, and you need to make sure your time is protected afterwards to give yourself chance to be kind to yourself; have a cup of tea and get ready to face the day again. It is important that you allow plenty of time to go through the following steps. I'd recommend at least an hour to do this.

Step 1 - *Start by writing down the things that you want to change, concentrating on the limiting beliefs that have been holding you back, i.e. 'I am not good enough', 'I am ugly', 'I am boring', 'I am fat'. I'd probably choose no more than three to start with.*

Step 2 – *Next, write down the positive consequences of continuing to believe this about yourself. Repeat this for each belief. How is this belief helpful? You may find that you cannot think of much to write here, there may be nothing at all!*

Step 3 - *Then take each one in turn and write down the negative consequences of continuing to believe these things about yourself, and what may happen if you don't change. I know this bit will feel painful but remember that's the point. Think about the future. If you keep believing that you are not good enough or if you keep abusing your body in this way, what's the worst that could happen? Really think about what your life could be like if you are still doing these things five years from now. Has this had an impact on your relationships? What do you look like? What job are you doing? How do you feel?*

Step 4 – *Spend a few moments with your eyes closed and really try to visualise what life will be like in five years' time if you don't change. If difficult emotions are emerging try not to push them away, imagine turning up a dial and increase the intensity of them, so that they feel as though they're going to burst through your chest.*

Step 5 *- When you have got a clear image in your head as to how your life might be, fast forward another five years and imagine what your life would be like in ten years' time. I know this is hard but try and persevere. Again, spend a couple of minutes sitting with these emotions and feel the pain.*

Step 6 *– When you're ready, gently and slowly open your eyes. Look around you, take in your surroundings. Ground yourself using the techniques I mentioned earlier.*

The difficult part of this exercise can be the realisation that you didn't really need to use your imagination or make anything up when thinking about how your life could be. That it could actually happen if things don't change. I imagine you have realised that holding on to these negative beliefs is just not healthy and is not going to be helpful to you or your future.

So, it's time to let them go, because do you know what? They are bullsh*t! Our beliefs aren't necessarily a reflection of reality; they're not true. I imagine you could think of a million reasons that counter these beliefs. I imagine you can think of a million ways in which you ARE good enough? The thing is, you've learnt these negative beliefs over the years by comparing yourself to others and taking on things others have said. Are you ready to unlearn them?

Step 7 *– Next, I want you to take your pen and paper again and write down the beliefs you want to have. Sometimes they are just the opposite of the limiting ones. For example, 'I am good enough', 'I am loveable', 'I am a good person', 'I am beautiful'. To learn these new beliefs on an unconscious level, repetition is essential. Say these to* *yourself everyday as part of your 'Hour of Power'; on your journey to work; while brushing your teeth. Just keep saying them!*

Step 8 – *Take these new, empowering beliefs and use them in the next exercise – The Ring of Power.*

Please know, this is one of the most difficult exercises I've done on my self-discovery journey, but it's one of the things that really gave me a kick up the bottom to change.

Please make sure that you take extra good care of yourself after doing this exercise as you may feel a bit fragile. Take an extra long bath, visit a friend, get an early night – whatever it is that you do to be kind to yourself.

Ring of power

Remember I said that you need to associate enough pain or pleasure to the thing that you want to change? Well, this is the pleasure part! This is a lovely exercise to do following the last one.

For this, you need to find a quiet spot where you can sit without being interrupted for ten minutes.

First, close your eyes and make sure that you are comfortable. Take steady breaths in and out and get into a relaxed, calm state. With your eyes closed, create a picture in your mind of the following...

Far in the distance, you can see a bright, white light shining up from ground, all the way to the sky. As you take a step closer and squint your eyes, you can see that the light is in the shape of a circle and, inside the circle, you can see a person standing in the middle.

Take a few, slow steps towards the light and as you look again you recognise the person. It's YOU! But you look different! You look happy, healthy and you are waving!

You can't quite believe your eyes and you feel as though you want to get closer to have a better look at this other you. You start to walk closer. As you do, you can see that the new you is the perfect weight; they're wearing the perfect clothes; they're dancing around and smiling as if they have not got a care in the world! They look confident and comfortable in their own skin, and they are not bothered what anyone else thinks because they're happy with who they are. They believe they are good enough; that they're beautiful; that they deserve happiness. They believe they are worth loving and have lots to offer the world. They look after themselves as they truly love themselves and make self-care their priority,

You take a few more steps closer but pause when you get to the ring of light on the floor. You suddenly have an overwhelming feeling *that you want to jump into the circle to be with the new you. Count down slowly in your head ...3 ....2 ...1 ... then hop/step/jump into the circle. Embrace the new you, jump around and breathe in what it would feel like to be like that. Turn up the positive emotion you're feeling so that it feels as though you're going to burst with joy. **This can be you! THIS IS YOU!***

As with the pain exercise, you may have noticed that it didn't take much of your imagination to create these positive images. That's because it isn't as far away as you think. The only thing that was different between the pain and pleasure exercise is what you believed about yourself. That's it! Every time you start to say or feel something negative about yourself, I want you to say, "That's bullsh*t!!!" Because it is! You now know that thinking in that negative way is only going to be harmful to you so take control of your thoughts and change them for something positive and empowering. For example, I might doubt whether I've made a positive parenting decision and start to feel as though I am a bad mum. When I notice myself slipping down this negative slope, I stop myself. Say, "That's bullsh*t!" and say, "I am a good enough mum. I am doing my best. I am loved". And for good measure, slip in at the end..."and I'm Claire f**king Reeves!"

I believe in you, even if you don't believe in yourself yet. If you apply the techniques and strategies in this book, commit to make small changes and apply them to your life consistently....you can become the person in the ring.

Remember...your destiny is truly in your hands.

"What you think, you become. What you feel, you attract. What you imagine, you create."

BUDDHA

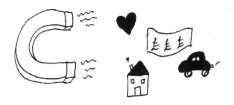

Make new friends

The people who we spend the most time with can have a big impact on our emotions, health and the beliefs we have about ourselves. When you're creating your new life, it's important to consider who you have in your support network and who you're spending time with. If you're surrounded by negative, narrow-minded, demotivated people then be careful, because they can rub off on you.

I'm not saying that you should ditch all your friends or that you need to cut anyone out, but it might be worth thinking about where you might be able to make friends with like-minded and positive people. If you spend time with friends with higher standards and that you aspire to be like, you will also find yourself naturally raising your standards. For example, if all your current friends drink heavily and don't take care of themselves, it can make it harder for you to sustain the changes you want to make, especially if there's pressure from your friends.

I don't drink anymore and my friends know this, but the amount of times I have been poured a glass of something or been told, "Go on, have one, it won't hurt you". Whereas, if you make friends with people that are also into fitness, meditation and that value self-care, it will be much easier to stay motivated and on track. Don't get rid of your old friends. Friends are a rare and special gift but look for others too – add to your circle – the old friends will get used to the new you soon. If they don't... well, were they really your friend after all?

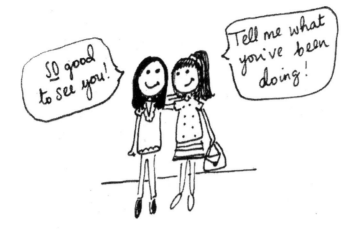

Remember...who you spend your time with is who you become.

Everyday problem-solving

Everyday life is tough. Just keeping on top of everything at home and work, at times, can feel like a battle. As adults, we have so many responsibilities and so many things to remember (especially if you're a parent!). When the boys told me they really wanted to take sandwiches to school instead of having school dinners, it nearly tipped me over the edge! I remember thinking, "This is yet another thing that I have to do/organise/ remember!" It felt like such a big deal as I was already run off my feet in a morning trying to get myself ready; get their uniforms ready; make my lunch for the day; pack their school bags. The list was endless and, needless to say, mornings were incredibly stressful, leading to me getting snappy and impatient – not a great way to start the day for anyone!

One day I stopped and thought about all the things that added extra stress to my life and thought about how I might be able do those things more efficiently and quickly. Just making minor alterations to my day made a big difference. I started listening to the boys read while I was straightening my hair; I made the sandwiches for the following day while I was making dinner and waiting for it cook; I tested the boys on their spellings and times tables whilst driving to school; I did my daily positive Facebook post whilst bouncing on the trampoline. Combining the jobs significantly cut down on the time I spent doing things, freeing up time to have more cuddles with the boys before school instead of moaning at them and rushing them out the door.

Finding simple solutions to my minor stresses made everything feel easier! Dr Rangan Chatterjee, in his book 'The Stress Solution', explains how these little stresses or 'micro-stresses' can easily build up throughout the day. Spending ten minutes preparing your lunch or getting your clothes ready the night before work can really help. It's one less thing to think about. Remember, the start of your day has a massive impact on the how it will pan out. If you can stay calm, organised and stress-free in the first couple of hours, you're much more likely to have a day that will follow on from this. Sometimes the solutions to the micro-stresses aren't obvious and you may need to think outside the box or enlist some help but there are solutions to most problems if you look hard enough.

I wonder...what are the little things in your day that stress you out?

Tidy house, tidy mind

We want your days to be filled with magic instead of stress and I don't think there is anything more stressful than not being able to find something. Losing things definitely triggers my inner rage! My husband is the worst for this. His version of tidying is putting things in the nearest drawer or cupboard rather than the ones they actually live in (it's making me feel tense as I'm writing this!). Although our house is tidy on the surface, if he needed something like his passport or latest pay slip, he would not have the foggiest. Of course, I respect his model of the world and accept that he has different priorities to me, but it still annoys me!

I truly believe in the phrase 'tidy house, tidy mind'. For me, when everything has its place; the shoe cupboard is tidy and my paperwork is filed properly, I can rest and sleep easy. I am not saying that I am the tidiest or cleanest person on the planet, but I do love a good sort out. I get great pleasure and a sense of achievement when sorting out my wardrobe or tidying my kitchen cupboards. When I can stand back and see the progress I've made, I feel in control and on top of life!

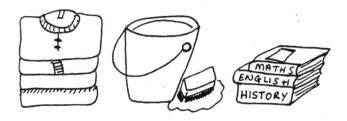

To create a life of order instead of chaos, think about how you can keep your things tidy. Maybe set yourself a task each week of sorting out a different cupboard or getting rid of clutter in a particular room. Be ruthless and bin anything you no longer need, or better yet, donate your unwanted things to a charity shop or clothes bank.

Remember...clutter in your physical space will create clutter in your mind.

Change or die!

I find it extremely important to set myself goals so that I have something to work towards and something to focus my energy on. Making progress, changing and growing are essential in life. Tony Robbins says that the day you stop growing and progressing is the day you die! You need to keep your brain and your body active to keep it working. You've heard the saying, *'If you don't use it, you lose it'*. It's so true. I am always challenging myself to learn new things and more importantly learn new things about myself, so that every day I can become the best version of me. People think that achieving goals brings you satisfaction. It obviously does, but not as much as the bit before that. When you are *making progress*, you feel in control, more mentally fit and often, immensely proud of yourself.

What changes do you want to make in your life? How are you going to get there?

Remember...progress equals happiness.

In summary...

*Nothing changes, if nothing changes. Changing your mindset, managing your emotions, feeling better about yourself and caring for your body are all great steps to creating your new life and your magical days. However, if you don't take action then the progress you make will be limited. The best way to make changes is to take **immediate massive action**. Instead of just saying, one day I'd like to run a marathon or I'm thinking about joining a weight loss class – book the marathon and contact the consultant of the weight loss class – TODAY!*

The sooner you can take action after making a decision, the more likely you will be to achieve that goal. Do it now before you have time to talk yourself out of it. Just do it! You need to set the wheels in motion as soon as possible. When you take massive action and step out of your comfort zone, things will naturally start to come together. Opportunities will appear, you will feel luckier as the Universe starts to align everything to help you to get to your destination. Magical days and a wonderful life are there for the taking. If you want it badly enough, you'll make it happen.

You can be who you want to be and do what you want to do, if you believe you can. I love the quote, 'If you think you can, or think you can't – you're right' (Henry Ford). If you believe in your goals and your reasons for changing, then you'll make it happen. If you don't think it is possible then it won't. The power of the mind is a wonderful thing.

With your new-found confidence, empowering beliefs and compelling goals, you are ready to take on the world!

A LAST LITTLE PIECE
OF ADVICE...

No matter how well you take care of yourself mentally and physically, you will have blips along the way and feel as though all your hard work has been for nothing. I have been there many times! What I have learnt is that once you start this journey, you can never go back to where you were. It's impossible. You won't be the same person. You can't unknow the things you've learnt. You will still have good days and bad days. I know I do. That's just life. That's being human. If you do feel stuck on your journey or lose motivation, don't worry. The worst thing you can do is beat yourself up about it. Show yourself patience and kindness and know that you'll get back to it when you're feeling better.

It has taken you a long time to create the unhealthy habits and negative beliefs that you've had. You've probably been doing the same thing for many years. You're not going to change overnight. This is a process of learning, and with any learning, mistakes need to be made for the lessons to really sink in. Whatever the blip, whatever the problem – remember to breathe. This will get you through it. Concentrating on your breathing will calm your mind and allow space in your brain to figure out what you need to do. It's in the quiet that you'll find the answers. And I want you to know, you already have the answers.

Even if you don't feel any different, have faith that what you're doing is working. If you're consistently taking care of your body and your mind, you will feel better. There will be days when things get too much and your emotions are over-whelming and clouding your judgement. Remember that nothing lasts forever – those emotions will pass, as will the tough days. Some days you might have to write off as being rubbish. As long as you make a conscious effort to start again when you're better, that's OK. Just take one day at a time. Concentrate on how you're going to make today the best it can be and how you can love yourself today.

Also, be aware that you're constantly changing and what works for you now may not work for you in a few months' time. So to continue to get to where you want to be and live the magical life that you want, you need to be flexible and adapt. Try something different until you find what fits.

There was something that I wasn't prepared for when I started my journey of change, and that was how other people reacted. There were very few people that seemed pleased when I started to change. My close family didn't like it at all when I started saying, "No" and no longer dropping everything to be at their beck and call. I was no longer meeting their needs, by focussing on my own. I don't blame them. They must have been incredibly confused because the Claire they knew seemed to be disappearing before their eyes, and I imagine it felt quite un-settling. Some unpleasant things were said to me as I started to put my needs first. I was called 'selfish', I was 'over-sensitive', I'd 'changed' (with an accusatory tone)', 'I needed to put my children first for once'. It made me doubt everything I was trying to do. I felt as though I was being a really horrible person. Luckily, I had my husband there to reassure me and encourage me to carry on taking care of myself. Changing was a painful process for us all to go through. We all needed time to adapt. Colleagues found it difficult to adapt also, as I rocked up with my weird, green smoothies, declaring I was a vegan, who no longer drank alcohol and only drank water or green tea! I imagine from the outside the changes I was making seemed quite drastic. They felt right to me though and still do.

I want you to know that the people who truly care about you will adapt, they'll come around and you never know, your new-found healthy, positive lifestyle may rub off on them. My husband has taken on board a lot of the things he's seen me do (apart from giving up meat, which would never happen in a million years!); I now have friends that have turned vegan/vegetarian and drink green tea despite being coffee addicts. Some have even started running. The biggest change I've noticed is in my relationships with my family now that everything has settled. Because I am more open with them about how I feel and because I express my gratitude more frequently, they do the same with me. My relationships have strengthened because of my new boundaries and honesty.

Some relationships will not strengthen though, and you have to be prepared to let go of anyone that sucks your energy and makes you feel bad about yourself. Don't be surprised if people make horrible comments if you lose weight or succeed in something new. Your success will bring out other people's insecurities. Your achievements will be reminders of the changes they need to make. Don't let anyone else's shadow dull your sparkle. This is your time to shine!

Whatever happens along the way, I want you to remember...

You are not responsible for how other people feel. You are only responsible for your emotions and creating a life that you are happy with.

Right then...I've officially shared with you everything I know! I imagine though, that by the time this book is printed, there would be many more things that I could add because I'm always learning about myself and how I can help others. Self-improvement is a lifelong project. There's always more to learn.

Remember how important you are. Change one or two things

at a time. Have blips but don't give up. Do it for you, because no-one else will.

The only thing left to do is...

GO FOR IT!!!!

Start creating your magical days <u>TODAY</u>!

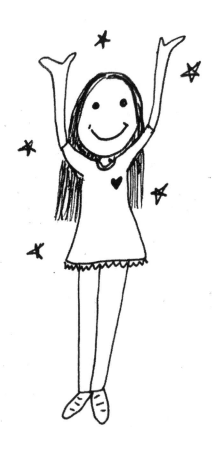

I wish you all the luck in the world as you begin your journey towards calmness and contentment.

Big love,

Claire

xxx

ACKNOWLEDGEMENT

A massive thank you to my beautiful and incredibly talented friend, Anne Austwick, for providing the illustrations for my book. We've known each other for more than half our lives, we've been through the good, bad and the ugly and I'm so grateful that you could be a part of this too. Big love forever Fanny.

To my wonderful but amazingly quirky family. I love you. Thank you for being there for me but also providing me with the experiences you have that have helped me to grow, learn and change. I wouldn't be doing what I'm doing without you.

ABOUT THE AUTHOR

Claire Reeves

Claire is a Psychotherapist and Master NLP Mindset Coach with a thriving private practice. She has always had a passion for helping others and a fascination with behavioural science. Claire has a degree in Psychology and is a former primary school teacher, as well as a Child Advocate and Service Manager for volunteers at a sexual abuse and rape advice centre.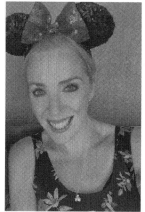

Using her integrative training and own personal experience of mental health issues, Claire's passion for helping others to overcome personal barriers in order to create their best life shines through.

Claire lives with her husband and two children. When she's not counselling, coaching or mummin', you will find her reading, running or singing along to Disney.

To connect with Claire or to find out more about her work, visit her website www.clairereeves.org.uk or email her at clairereevescounselling@gmx.com.